1/2016

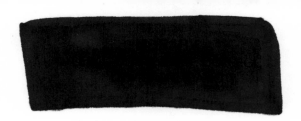

WITHDRAWN

THE
FUTURE
OF MENTAL
HEALTH

THE
FUTURE
OF MENTAL
HEALTH

Deconstructing
the Mental
Disorder
Paradigm

Eric Maisel

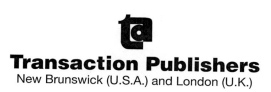

Transaction Publishers
New Brunswick (U.S.A.) and London (U.K.)

Library of Congress Catalog Number: 2015016606
ISBN: 978-1-4128-6261-5 (cloth); 978-1-4128-6249-3 (paper)
eBook: 978-1-4128-6204-2
Printed in the United States of America

Library of Congress Cataloging-in-Publication Data

Maisel, Eric, 1947-
    The future of mental health : deconstructing the mental disorder paradigm / Eric Maisel.
        pages cm
    Includes bibliographical references and index.
    ISBN 978-1-4128-6261-5 -- ISBN 978-1-4128-6249-3 -- ISBN 978-1-4128-6204-2 1. Mental health. 2. Mental health services. 3. Mental health planning. I. Title.
    RA790.6.M25 2015
    362.2--dc23
                                                                    2015016606

For Ann, as always

Contents

Introduction

This book is intended for four audiences: mental health professionals, individuals suffering with emotional distress, parents of children who find themselves pulled into the world of the mental health establishment, and interested lay people who would like to learn more about our current crisis in mental health service provision, its roots, and its remedies.

For mental health professionals, I'll paint a picture of the movement they may want to make away from the current misguided practice of "diagnosing and treating mental disorders." I'll show a way toward a wiser, truer, more humane, and more effective practice that focuses on a sufferer's complaints and problems, formed personality, life experiences, current circumstances, and existential realities rather than on "symptom pictures" and the mechanical, illegitimate application of mental disorder labels.

For current practitioners, this is a hard stance to take due to the demands of managed care, the power of drug companies, the need for insurance reimbursement, inadequate and inappropriate training, a desire to maintain a chimerical prestige based on putative expertise, and their position of being firmly embedded inside a deceitful system. I will also propose a new mental health helper, someone I call a "human experience specialist," who, not stuck and pressured in these ways, might offer new, better help to sufferers.

For individuals who are suffering, I want them to understand all of the following. First, they must realize that emotional distress, even severe emotional distress, is natural. It is not desirable, but it is natural. There is a vast difference, as different as conceptualizing the earth as flat versus round, between a brain being broken and a human being despairing. Right now we are operating with the "flat earth" version. It is your job as a suffering person not to accept some easy-to-swallow label that seems to explain your struggle but in reality explains nothing. Your job is to step to the plate as an investigator of your own painful situation.

Second, I want people who are suffering to understand steps that can help them: how it can help them to refuse to be labeled a patient; how it can help them to understand the difference between "psychiatric medication" and prescribed chemicals with powerful effects (effects they may in fact sometimes want); how it can help them to dispute the idea that "normal" and "abnormal" are sensible words; how it can help them to learn about institutions and communities of care that are radically different from the usual in-patient warehousing; and more. This is not the sort of help offered in self-help books. This is "meta" help: I want you to step back, survey the landscape, and better understand the basics.

As for parents, you have a new responsibility. Not only are you obliged to feed, clothe, and care for your children; not only is it your job to shower them with love, kindness and respect; not only is it your responsibility to teach them life skills and help them make sense of the world. You have a new job as well: watching out that you and your children aren't victimized by the current mental health system and its wanton mental disorder labeling practices. It is your job to educate yourself about how the mental health establishment operates and decide if you believe its rationales for wanting to affix a mental disorder label to your child and begin him or her on so-called medication to treat a so-called disorder.

I also hope that interested laypeople, who may or may not be currently suffering, will nevertheless find these ideas eye-opening and may even be provoked to activism. There are many worthy causes to champion in life, and there is only so much that any individual can do. But by the same token, the emotional and mental health of our species—and especially of our children—is a cause worthy enough to rise to the top of any activist list. Your useful activism might be as simple as saying out loud, "Does it really make sense that a five-year-old might find himself on two, three, or four psychiatric medications? Really?" Even just some wide-eyed, noisy wondering might start to make a difference.

I would like to see a mental health revolution, and I intend to describe what the contours of that revolution might look like. In that regard, this is a manifesto, a cry for change, a plea on behalf of helpless children being fed pills at the drop of a diagnosis, and a demand that sufferers receive different and better help than that currently provided by the mental health establishment. Is such a revolution possible in the face of our entrenched ways, the power of invested parties, and a deep, culture-wide acceptance of the "mental disorder" model? Well, even kings have been toppled!

I am certainly not the only one writing about these ideas. In the suggested reading list at the end, you will find books with titles like *The Myth of Mental Illness*, *Toxic Psychiatry*, *The Myth of the Chemical Cure*, and many others. For half a century, a minority opinion has announced that mental health service provision has been corrupted by a pair of falsehoods, that "mental disorders" (as opposed to human suffering) exist, and that the way to treat these "mental disorders" is to act like they are akin to physical disorders and medicate the sufferer or act like they are not physical at all but "psychological" in nature and treatable through "expert talk."

Many people have previously decried these as corrupt, flat-earth approaches to helping people who are suffering with mental and emotional pain. But for a variety of reasons, including the promulgation of a new mental health labeling catalogue called the DSM-5 (the Diagnostic and Statistical Manual of the American Psychiatric Association, Fifth Edition, which has taken a great deal of fire even from entrenched mental health professionals), the rapid increase of the labeling of children with so-called mental disorders, and the ever more brazen marketing by pharmaceutical companies of chemicals for every possible human difficulty, this is perhaps a new moment.

Let me say a word about the following. In this book, I argue that our current mental health practices are faulty. But I also make it quite clear, and spend a whole chapter on this subject, that difficult people are genuinely difficult. A dangerously "crazy" person can be a serious threat to others, and society has a legitimate right to protect itself from dangerous people. It is an issue up for serious debate as to whether we want to use chemicals to control dangerous folks.

I do not want my basic argument, that these chemicals are not actually medicine and that what is going on is nothing like "diagnosing and treating mental disorders," to become hijacked by natural concerns about what to do with "crazy" people who jump White House fences, behead their neighbor, or engage in school shootings. I am giving them no license! And in fact, we will have an easier time trying to discern what type of help such individuals need once we clearly understand what is *not* being done now.

Maybe these are ideas whose time has come. Perhaps the billions of people worldwide who suffer from emotional and mental distress may be helped by realizing they haven't been infected with a "mental illness virus" that a chemical can cure and that they haven't succumbed to some mere "psychological issue." Rather, they are having a painful whole-being reaction to the nameable, predictable problems of living. That would amount to an earth-shattering change, a genuine paradigm shift, and it would begin the process of helping sufferers finally reduce their emotional pain.

1

Our Human Experience

In our current environment, where the answer to every life difficulty is a mental disorder label and a pill instead of wise counsel, your mental health is at greater risk than ever. And your mental health matters! How much joy and pleasure can you get out of life, how well can you manifest your life purposes, and how likely is it that life will feel meaningful to you if you are stewing, despairing, seething, or worrying? Your mental health is precious! And while life comes with real difficulties that threaten that mental health, you aren't left stranded without answers or resources. There is help.

Woven into the following discussion is a picture of a worldview that includes the dangers of accepting the current mental health labeling system, the help currently available, what future help might look like, and what it means to be human. It is a worldview that may liberate and motivate you. You will relearn many things that you already know: that life is difficult, that emotional distress is inevitable, and that personality is a mix of the intractable and the improvable. By the end of our discussion, I hope that you will experience a breath of fresh air.

You may also be interested in the new profession that I describe in these pages: human experience specialist. This profession does not currently exist and quite possibly never will—unless, of course, you and others see to its creation. The headline is that this book may help you both personally and professionally. It may help you professionally especially if you are already a therapist, counselor, social worker, or other front line worker who would like to shift your focus from "diagnosing and treating mental disorders" to something more human and helpful.

Let's begin in what may seem like too obvious a way: by reminding ourselves that human beings have human experiences. On the face of it this sounds ludicrous. Who doesn't know this? You know exactly what it feels like to be rejected, to hate your job, to need to divorce your mate, to feel suddenly overwhelmed by some trifle. You know what it's like to have tax season arrive again, to worry about that spot on your skin, to not like what your son just said to you, to not much like your own personality. Why would I need to remind you that human beings have human experiences?

Well, you need reminding because the mental health establishment is vehemently opposed to this view. Since you are bombarded and affected by the view that there is some lovely, unreal, pain-free state called "normal" and scores of "mental disorders" that blow in through the open window to threaten that fictional "normal"—a view promoted on every talk show and in every advertisement for so-called psychiatric medication—you may actually have lost your natural understanding that life is life.

Tens of millions of people have indeed lost this natural understanding, including the millions of parents of children who, at the first sign that their child is having a difficult time, willingly—even instantly—adopt the perspective that they have a "little patient" in the house. This movement from the reality of human experience to the unreality of "a mental disorder for every difficulty" has been fast-tracked to gospel—and you may have become one of its unwitting victims and co-conspirators. Let us start there, by reminding ourselves what life is like. Let's get our hands dirty in the human experience.

Holding Her Breath

During World War II, sixty million people died, more than 2.5 percent of the world's population. The Soviet Union alone lost between eighteen and twenty-four million lives. Germany lost between seven and nine million, upwards of 10 percent of its population. Europe's Jewish population was reduced by between five and six million, or 55 percent of European Jewry. A country like Portugal lost "only" fifty thousand souls, but those fifty thousand amounted to 10 percent of the Portuguese population.

Forget for a second about who was in the right and who was in the wrong. Rather, imagine a German youth of eighteen, a Russian youth of eighteen, a British youth of eighteen, an American Jewish youth of eighteen, a French youth of eighteen, a Japanese youth of eighteen. Think of the parents of each of these young men, parents, say, between forty and forty-five years old. Think of their grandparents. Think of their sisters, their younger brothers—think about everyone affected by that calamity.

To say that the "mental health" of all of these people was affected by the fact of a world conflagration is to make a bad joke. Affected, indeed!

It may have been the defining, pressing, most important matter on their radar, completely altering their lives and producing year upon year of unbearable stress. The whole world's population was "motivated" in drastically new ways—and unmotivated as well. How motivated would you have been to open up your grocery store each morning if you had to sell to your Nazis oppressors? How motivated would you have been to get out of bed if your city was under siege?

Psychology posits many "theories of motivation." These include an instinct theory of motivation (e.g., birds migrating), an incentive theory of motivation (e.g., external rewards), a drive theory of motivation (e.g., drink water when thirsty), an arousal theory of motivation (e.g., cure boredom with an action movie), a humanistic theory of motivation (e.g., self-actualization), and more. To vote for any one of these—or some combination of them, or all of them in the aggregate—is to make a fundamental mistake.

The mistake is the way that these theories exclude the human experience. We aren't machines functioning or not functioning in mechanical ways. We are human beings who think, feel, live, and organize our experiences in existential and psychological ways. The problem isn't that all of these theories have nothing to say. The problem is that this way of thinking prevents us from understanding human beings. The human being is almost always lost when a theory is proposed, whether that theory is psychoanalytic, cognitive-behavioral, or, as in the "mental disorder" model, pseudo-medical.

Think of the mother of that young soldier. It doesn't matter whether he is German, Russian, French, British, or Japanese. Her son goes off to war, and he has, say, a 20 or 30 percent chance of dying. For the years that he is away, she is fundamentally not motivated at all, though, of course, she still drinks water when she is thirsty, plays the lottery in the hopes of a windfall, and shows up at work to receive her paycheck.

She is "motivated" in all the textbook ways—she gets to work, she buys lottery tickets, she drinks water, she has sex—but her reality is that she is holding her breath. If you ask her why she is having headaches, stomachaches, sleep problems, an inability to orgasm, and sudden crying fits, she may well tell you, "I am waiting for my son to come home." Should we really stand for a psychiatrist answering this with, "I have a pill for that mental disorder!"? Should we really stand for a psychotherapist exclaiming, "Oedipal issues!"? We should not. Our new helper of the future, our new human experience specialist, would begin by replying simply and humanly, "I know."

Our new helper would say to her, "I understand. I know that you are holding your breath, and I know why you are holding your breath. I want to make the following couple of suggestions, neither of which will fundamentally change your situation. Your fundamental situation is that you are waiting, that you are holding your breath, and that you are scared to death. I completely understand. But I do have a couple of suggestions to make. Shall we look at them?"

This isn't psychiatry or psychotherapy, it isn't mentoring, coaching, or counseling, and it isn't friendship. It requires a new category of helper, a person not bound to establish goals and cheerlead like a coach; not bound, like mental health counselors, psychologists, and psychotherapists, to buy our current "diagnosing and treating of mental disorders" model; not bound, like a psychiatrist, to dispense pills; not bound, like a cleric, to lecture about what gods demand; not bound to ignore a human being's real, pressing, and defining experiences and circumstances. There would be no "diagnosing" and no "treating." Instead, there would be a human interaction in the context of calamity.

And who isn't in the middle of calamity? Forget about world wars. What is it like for the quarter million women diagnosed with breast cancer each year and the one in eight women threatened by it? What is it like for a gay youth in a fundamentalist town? What is it like for a workingman or workingwoman living in a tract home in Ft. Worth, Queens, or Dayton? What is it like for a writer with no publisher, a painter with no gallery, a musician with no gigs? What is it like for an obese man or woman with no sex life? What is it like for the millions who hate their jobs, the millions with no job, the millions who cringe when their mate enters the room, or the millions who have aged into invisibility?

Despite all of this mental stress, distress, and misery, we are supposed to stand "mentally healthy," as if life were a lark and as if sweet smiles were not only our birthright, but also our obligation. Why should we be smiling? Why should we be "mentally healthy," whatever that phrase is supposed to mean? For the whole history of our species, until very recently, even your drinking water could kill you. In our age of good drinking water—which is only a reality for a small percentage of our species—we have had world wars and nuclear weapons to contend with. And what is life like for someone living under a dictator, where you can vanish for speaking? And how pleasant, for that matter, is your own seething mind, packed with worries, regrets, resentments, and to-do lists? Why should you be mentally healthy?

Nevertheless, you are supposed to keep smiling. You are supposed to stay positive. No matter that every human right must continually be fought for. No matter that in this modern age of plenty, which advertising tells us comes with beautiful homes, beautiful cars, and beautiful bodies, insomnia is epidemic, obesity is epidemic, sadness is epidemic, and meaninglessness is epidemic. You must not notice the machinations of the powerful. None of that should affect your mental health. You must not notice your aging, your illnesses, or your mortality. None of that should affect your mental health. You may not even look in the mirror and announce that you might strive to be a better person. No, none of that!

Against this backdrop of great difficulty; stresses to our system; dangers as real as wars, famines, and pestilences; and a mind that races of its own accord and seethes over injustices and indignities, has grown a mental health establishment that takes none of that into account. It acts as if our baseline is "mental health" and that deviations from that unreal, made-up baseline are "mental disorders" or "mental diseases." It calls the warehousing of distressed and difficult people, people who are no picnic and who are having no picnic, the "institutionalization of the mentally ill." Its psychiatrists spend fifteen minutes with patients, not exploring human matters but prescribing and regulating chemicals. That is where we are today.

That establishment creates countless labels for human distress, individual differences, natural reactions to painful stressors, and socially unacceptable behavior, and it announces that this hungry, sad boy has a "clinical depression," as if something blew in the window and into his brain. It says that this unhappy, bitterly unfulfilled woman has a "clinical depression," as if her husband despising her wasn't as real as bricks. It says that this arthritic old man whom his children have long since stopped visiting has a "clinical depression," as if it were really a lark to sit in a wheelchair in the corridor of a nursing home from morning till night.

It takes no account of the extent to which human beings fail and how much failing hurts. For every PGA champion there are thousands of golf pros and would-be golf pros chastising themselves for not playing well enough, down on themselves for their lack of talent, their lack of discipline, and their lack of success. For every NBA star there are millions of young men completely thwarted in their dreams of rising out of the hell of tenements, drugs, gangs, and violence, and who at some very early age throw in the towel and live a life of menace. For every country western singer who wins multiple Grammys there are legions of waitresses in dives all across America singing along to the music they wish they were singing on *The Voice* as they wipe up coffee spills and scrape dried eggs off table tops. We fixate on that PGA champion, that NBA star, and that celebrity singer—each of whom, by the way, is having his or her own meltdown, as any tabloid will tell you—and not on the "boring" ordinary people with failed dreams and bad lives who are supposed to keep smiling.

Ignoring our species' continuous history of difficulty and ongoing difficulties, difficulties that can be increased any day of the week by a new war, a new plague, a new drought, a glacial winter, or just the continuous barking of a neighbor's dog, the mental health establishment, with your willing participation, has contrived to make all of these difficulties "abnormal" and, as a result, profitable to them. When you get very sad because life feels horrible or very anxious because everything, from your bills to your mate, feels threatening, they tell you that you have a "mental disorder." Either you nod your head in agreement and accept their pills and their "expert talk," or you announce your defiant disagreement and . . . then what? If you do not accept the mental health establishment's way of viewing your pain, and if that pain remains, what will you do then?

In addition to the genuine help currently available, which we will discuss, it would be wonderful if in the future you could speak with a new type of professional: a human experience specialist. Countless psychotherapists, violating the letter of their license and not at all happy "diagnosing and treating mental disorders," already function as human experience specialists—and could be converted over to this new category easily, so ready are they to be untethered from the current untenable system. This is, of course, what psychotherapy should have been all along—a human experience specialty—rather than a pseudo-medical profession where even master's level professionals assert that they have "patients."

Right now, change is tremendously difficult. Just follow the money. Follow the prestige, the power, the insider connections, the holding of hands, and the washing of hands. Follow the intense ties throughout the establishment in all of its colorful garb: pharmaceutical companies, academics, hospitals, HMOs, mental institution executives, courts, expert classes, jailers, the advertising industry, politicians, bureaucracies, talk show hosts. A great many people are invested in taking money from you—and taking your very freedom—the second you complain of some difficulty. Against this reality, it is hard to propose that human experience start to count for something.

Let me add that the practice of prescribing psychiatric medication should not completely vanish. There is a profound difference between chemicals with powerful effects, which is what psychiatrists prescribe, and psychiatric medication, which is what they claim to be prescribing. The rationale for calling them "medicine" presumes the presence of diseases and disorders that have never been proven to exist. They were created around committee tables and ought to be disbelieved. However, some sufferers may want the effects of these chemicals, and for that reason psychiatrists would still be needed. We'll return to this important question of which parts of the current mental health system are worth keeping. For now, let me repeat that if we forget that human beings have human experiences, we do so at our own peril.

Genuine Not Knowing

The reality of the human experience is known to each of us, just so long as we don't forget it. What we don't understand is man himself. Man is the elephant in the room. We don't really understand why he so easily goes off to war—a good war, a bad war, any war. We don't really understand why he can't stop smoking cigarettes even though his life depends on him stopping. We don't really understand why, having been beaten as a child and pledging with all his heart not to beat his own children, he nevertheless does so. We just don't understand the why of human beings.

We don't know to what extent man comes with a blueprint, what exactly to make of the idea of "genetic predispositions," or why a cloud passing in front of the sun can make him feel so very sad. What we don't know is vastly greater than what we do know. It is very hard for people to accept the truth that we don't know what we need to know about man—and that quite possibly we will never know what we need to know. It may prove easier to learn about the distant reaches of the universe, the beginning of time, and the inside of atoms than about what makes man tick. This is a hard truth to swallow.

But we must start there, announcing how little we know. Our "mental health experts" aren't very expert. Neither past nor current thinkers and practitioners know what is going on "inside" human beings. Brain scans will never get at why an environmental activist pickets against nuclear energy one year and then sees it as man's best hope for clean energy the next. There is no brain scan, present or future, that can paint a picture of personality, consciousness, or the internal conversations that human beings hold. One of the calamities of the current system is the way in which a show of knowing is made.

Let me hasten to add that the critics of the current system do not know what is going on "inside" any better than do the established "experts." The critics likewise have only their own ungrounded opinions. For instance, Thomas Szasz, a well-known opponent of contemporary psychiatric practices, proposed that what we are seeing with disturbed people are not symptoms of illness but human beings angling for what they want via playacting. Szasz observed that as soon as a particular game became socially unacceptable—say, for women to act "hysterically"—that "mental illness" simply vanished. When fainting fell out of fashion, women simply stopped fainting. Szasz's ideas are provocative and interesting, but who can really say? And how could we ever really know?

R. D. Laing, another critic of the current system, portrayed "mental disorders" rather more as breakthroughs than breakdowns: episodes of a kind of battle for health, clarity, and spiritual relief that required a self-directed plunge into darkness. Jung held a rather similar view. There are countless pictures one can paint as to what human beings look to be experiencing, feel compelled to do, or seem to will into existence. You can say anything about a human being without needing any proof—you can say that he is being bad, that he is being willful, that he is on a journey of transformation, that he has a genetic predisposition, that he has a complex, that he has an illness. In the absence of knowing, nothing is easier than saying.

These are our starting points: the reality of human experience and the reality of our not knowing. Take a vulnerable child—that is, any child—thrust that child into the hardness of life, add some extra difficulty for good measure, and then let that child burn with its billions of neurons ablaze like stars on fire. What will that child think and feel? Why would that child be happy? Content? Comfortable in his or her own skin? Why would a child stand fearless after experiencing all sorts of terrors: the terror of uncontrolled appetite, the terror of cruel humanity, the terror of unpaid bills, and the terror of empty hours? We do not know why people do what they do, but we know that they are human beings like us, that they have been hammered in the crucible of reality.

You would expect helping professionals to start there too. You would expect them to understand that a bored child might act out, that a beaten child might have trouble sleeping, that a person who has lost his or her business might feel defeated, that a person who grew up in a cult might have trouble confronting authority. You would expect professionals to understand these human things and take them into account before "diagnosing" and "treating." Yet the professionals' bible, the DSM-5, takes none of that into account. Their training takes none of that into account, and it is not their inclination to start doing so.

I would ask us to erase the blackboard, admit all that we do not know, and start with the genuine human experience, the one where it is hard to make small talk, hard to make meaning, hard to make friends, hard to make magic, hard to make a life that works. If we would only start there, flying in the face of the avid pill pushers and our ghastly game of pseudo-medicine, we might be able to ask certain questions forthrightly, questions like, "Given that pain and disappointment are coming, what can a human being do?"

If anyone can know the answer to a question like that as it pertains to you, mustn't that person be you? Isn't it reasonable to suppose that you must prove to be the expert about your own mental health, the only expert really, and that any mental health service provider you hire ought to be viewed as a collaborator in the process and not as the boss of it? If there are organic reasons for your distress—if, say, you have a brain tumor—then it's vital that you receive genuine medical help. But if the reasons for your distress are rooted in some boiling conflict, in the shadows of your own personality, in your despairing view of life, isn't it on your shoulders to become the expert of all that? Mustn't you carry that weight?

You must. You may not want to, but nevertheless you must. If we could take as our starting point that human beings like you and me find this world difficult, instead of starting from a place where there is something called "mental health" and some things called "mental disorders," then we would be telling a truth that we have always known but that has become submerged under an ocean of propaganda. You are a person of flesh and blood, someone who can smile, who has nightmares, who is completely unlike the picture of you painted by the mental health establishment. And ultimately you must carry the weight of life—and the weight of responsibility for dealing with life.

The future of mental health is also the future of your mental health. You can bank on your mental health being threatened. It may be threatened from the outside by calamities, indignities, and defeats. It may be threatened from the inside by festering wounds, painful conflicts, and unrealized dreams. Given that it will be threatened, what will you do?

9

I hope to provide you with some tentative answers. What, really, can be an "answer" to life? But even tentative answers can prove a blessing. I hope you experience them that way.

Let me summarize. We are confronted by several daunting truths:

- What is currently being provided by way of mental health services is below par. Much of it is downright fraudulent.
- The current system makes money, bestows prestige, and provides a power base for putative experts, leaving them with no particular incentive for change.
- We have very little understanding of what goes on "inside" human beings.
- Human beings are difficult in a variety of ways, including in their unwillingness to change and in their reluctance to collaborate, making it hard for even compassionate helpers.
- We have no "treatments" for emotional distress that mirror medical treatments since what we are "treating" is life.
- Our minimization of the reality of the human experience is entrenched, and that minimization makes itself felt everywhere.

Maybe these daunting challenges actually provide us with a unique opportunity to step back and start over. Starting from precisely where we are, mostly in the dark, how should we conceptualize emotional distress? What should we offer sufferers of emotional distress? What sensible distinctions can we make between one sort of distress and another? How can we help people help themselves deal with life? These are our questions. Some of my answers may surprise you. However, we have considerable ground to cover before we can get to suggestions and recommendations. We have a lot of housecleaning to do before we can bring in the new furniture.

2

The Naturalness of Distress

Our first piece of housecleaning is ridding ourselves of the false idea that distress is unnatural. Given that we have evolved into the exact creature that we are, nothing could be more natural than feeling sad, anxious, bored, overwhelmed, defeated, or otherwise distressed. I am saying nothing new here—this idea is a cornerstone of Buddhism, for instance—and yet its reality remains largely unacknowledged, either by individuals in distress or by those paid to help them. As a society, we treat distress as surprising and unnatural when it is instead completely predictable and natural.

Imagine that we were designed for a particular purpose (for example, to live happily, to serve dutifully, or for some other purpose conjured up by the mind of the designer). Then we would be a very different species. If our designer wanted us to sleep well, which might align with its purpose that we work hard each day in its service, then it would provide us with an accessible off switch that would allow us to turn ourselves off for eight hours and sleep blissfully. That would end our insomnia epidemic. If it wanted us to be happy, which might align with its purpose that we not question it and revolt, it would highly limit our consciousness to the consciousness of happy things.

If we are designed for a specific purpose, it would eliminate our experience of psychological pain, it would prevent us from reaching for hard-to-attain goals, and it would summarily end our "depression" epidemic. Our designer would not build us to become addicted. It would not build us to become bored. Unless it were an extremely sloppy designer, it would do a much better job of completely eliminating human distress so that its creatures could do a workmanlike job of fulfilling its purposes. Needing to give us just enough consciousness to perform certain tasks, it would give us no more than that.

But we are not designed. We show our lack of design and the realities of evolution in a million ways. The primary way we show our lack of design and our evolutionary history is in the area of mental distress.

A designed creature would not pester itself so much, not experience such lifelong harm from its early negative experiences, not have such poignant needs as meaning and life purpose, not operate so blindly and keep repeating mistakes, and not experience change in the direction of better mental health as so amazingly difficult.

Human beings, having evolved into the makeshift creature that we are, experience all of these distresses. We experience distress when we are treated unfairly. We experience distress when we look in the mirror and hate what we see. We experience distress when we don't get what we want. We experience distress when we contemplate death and the end of our existence. We experience distress when we are forced to toil pointlessly just to pay the rent. We experience distress when we want two contradictory things, like the opportunity to create and the opportunity to make a living. We experience distress when society orders us about, lies to us, closes us in, or demands that we act in certain ways. We experience distress if we are poor, if we are bored, and when our own thoughts attack us. A smartly designed creature would experience none of this. We do.

This is who we are. Relationships fail. We fail ourselves. Our entertainments don't amuse us. Our life purposes elude us, as does the experience of meaning. In our current mental health system, and woven throughout the history of theorizing about mental health and mental disorders, little or none of this basic evolutionary distress is taken into account. It is as if we have coveted and as a result created an image of a distress-free creature, an ideal human being who has never existed and never could exist. There is no ideal deer, one that has never had to flee from lions. There is no ideal giraffe, one that can pick up small objects at its feet. There is no ideal elephant, one able to squeeze into subcompacts. And there is no ideal human being, one who keeps smiling in the face of life's painful challenges. Nothing could be more fanciful or absurd—or so unhelpful—than to dream up such an unreal creature.

To say that these distresses are biological and psychological is to say nothing of moment. Everything human is biological and psychological. When we enjoy a party, it is biological and psychological. When we push aside the peas on our plate, it is biological and psychological. It adds nothing to the discussion of human affairs to call a phenomenon like distress biological or psychological unless we are very precise about what additional meanings we intend to add by saying that. If we intend to add some idea like "disorder" or "biological malfunction" or "psychological impairment," then we had better be ready and able to explain ourselves and prove our assertions. We will have more to say on this in later chapters.

These ordinary, predictable, and painful distresses are challenges to be handled and problems in need of attention. They are not disorders. Being human is not a disorder. For example, it is not a disorder to care about our fellow human beings and to also feel intensely self-interested. That is rather more a definition of being human than a disorder. Yet the conflict between humanist values and selfishness produces great distress in every smart, sensitive person. That resulting distress is poignant, painful, and even dreadful, but it is not the product of a disorder, a symptom of a disorder, or a marker of a disorder. It arises because we have evolved with exactly such contradictory motives.

Human beings are conflicted about whether to do the right thing or to do what we want to do. Our sense of right and wrong, bound up with knowledge of human rights history and endless information about a world of wrongs occurring daily, must contend with our desire for orgasms, gas-guzzling cars, easy entertainments, victories at games, and other features of our genetic self-interest. To have a conscience and to also be self-interested does not constitute a disorder. This is the sort of naturally occurring, nonpathological human distress that our future mental health service providers must be trained to address.

That we are conflicted this way, one day pledging to help starving children and the next day not caring about starving children at all, will not surprise this new mental health professional. I painted a picture in the last chapter of a mother whose son is off to war, whose inner life is organized around the dread that he will not return, and how she lives her life while holding her breath. Now consider another archetypal wartime figure: the Nazi commandant of Paris. On the one hand, and with no qualms whatsoever, he sends Jews to their death by the trainloads. On the other hand, and under great pressure not to ignore Hitler's direct order, he is nevertheless persuaded not to burn down Paris. His self-interest screams burn it down, since his wife and children are marked for execution if he ignores that order. Yet he refrains from giving the order.

The murderer and the savior can be one-and-the-same person. We have evolved into a creature that both cares about values and does not care about values. We have it in us to be greedy and generous—don't most robber barons end up donating to charity? We have it in us to be cruel and compassionate, deceitful and honest, sadistic and loving. The strain on the system that this never-ending conflict produces is no joke. But it is not a disorder. It is not a disorder for our genes to express themselves in ways that dismay us and even floor us. That kindly grandfather can also be an architect of genocide. We can fail ourselves in similar, if smaller, ways by having an affair that ruins our marriage, by finishing the milk rather than leaving a little behind, by being snide and sarcastic just because we are full of ourselves. That we are of two minds is not a brain disorder.

No body part here is malfunctioning. No brain scan can distinguish between a brain that will burn down Paris and one that will not. No brain scan can distinguish a brain that agrees to have an extramarital affair from one that refrains from the affair. These are not body part problems but species problems. Do we think that not wanting to shake hands is an arm problem? Is yelling at your mate a mouth problem? Is not liking what you see when you look at your art an eye problem? Is the anxiety you feel in the pit of your stomach a stomach problem? Why then do we think that feeling sad is a brain problem? Just because your sadness feels "located" in your skull, you must not make the assumption that something is wrong with your brain chemistry.

Now, if you can't shake hands because you do have an arm problem, that's another matter. Not wanting to shake hands is one thing. Not being able to shake hands is another thing. If there was any proof whatsoever that "mental disorders" or states like sadness were similar to a physical ailment, then we would be looking at a body part or a body system as the culprit. But there is zero proof that boredom, sadness, worry, doubt, despair, irritability, agitation, gloominess, anger, self-pestering, joylessness, frustration, or other human distresses are body part problems. Rather, there is a deep common sense understanding that they are not.

But what about the wilder "disorders" like the thing called "schizophrenia"? Surely that must be a body part problem. Well, nobody knows. With the thing called "schizophrenia" all of the following have been floated as the "breakage" causing the "illness": overactivity of the neural transmitter dopamine; serotonin issues; faulty metabolic brain processes; genetic predisposition; abnormalities in the structure or function of the brain; the "inappropriate connecting" of neurons during fetal development; and so on. But no one knows, and there is substantial evidence that "schizophrenia" is just a label we apply to a wide range of behaviors with no known common cause. We must not call a thing a brain problem if we do not know if it is. Until we know, we do not know.

In the "biological breakage" view, a person has not arrived at his current destination because of his reactions to life, the ways he has managed his stressors and his distress, the way his personality is expressing itself, or any willfulness on his part. Rather, something is physically wrong with him. Something biological has been visited on him. Is this true? No one currently knows, and in the absence of knowing we have decided to ignore the possibility that distress is the main culprit. We are "all in" on the guess that what is going on is a biological malfunction, as much because human beings are so difficult to deal with that we prefer to prescribe a pill and otherwise wash our hands of the matter. We will come back to this question of "breakage"—of its reality and of its utility as a metaphor—when we discuss cause and effect in human affairs.

The distress I've been describing is not a brain problem and not a body part problem. We are inclined to think that it is because human nature continually surprises us. We have only a muffled executive awareness and an inadequate system of remarking to ourselves that this or that natural thing has happened. Who doesn't know that not getting the bicycle you wanted as your Christmas present will hurt? Yet not getting it still hurts. Who doesn't know that discovering that your mate is cheating on you will hurt? Yet learning that terrible news still hurts. As a species, we can't seem to inoculate ourselves against painful experiences feeling painful. Because we can't inoculate ourselves, because that hurt surprises us each time and hurts each time, we inadvertently create a false picture of life: an enduring state of peace punctuated by diabolical jabs and blows. Yet the jabs and blows are just as natural as the peace.

Take another one of those jabs and blows and a great source of our distress: work. Work is absurd. The idea that we must spend half of our waking hours toiling at something just to pay the rent is horrible on the face of it. Yet people are somehow surprised that work causes them distress. They feel like a bad sport for pointing a finger at the absurdity of work. Presumably machines have no opinions about work, but why shouldn't a creature with consciousness, one that can imagine its life purposes and experience the difference between a meaningful time and a meaningless time, hate being subjected to all that meaningless toiling? What could be more natural than finding meaningless work distressing? Imagine decade after decade of it! Yet every child is primed to picture some wonderful work that is supposed to occupy him for a lifetime. Children are not instructed that work will come in two flavors: meaningful work and meaningless work. Most work will amount to the latter.

Society needs the vast majority of its workforce to engage in unrewarding jobs. That those jobs may prove unrewarding and create chronic distress is never mentioned. No one points a finger or has the inclination to bother, in large part because there are no alternatives and no remedies. It isn't that twelve people sitting around a table at universal headquarters collude to agree that drones are needed for the system no matter how that affects their mental health. There is no conspiracy of that sort. Rather, it is in the nature of our species, another proof of our evolutionary roots, that work is not questioned. Neither bosses, who need employees, nor employees, who need jobs, are inclined to point a finger at the indignity of meaningless work. So the game is played generation after generation as workers despair—and suffer the added indignity of feeling prohibited from denouncing the very idea of work.

Mental health professionals play along and say nothing. Only a cynical mental health professional would dare argue that spending a lifetime engaged in meaningless work for the sake of paying the rent wouldn't sadden, stress, and even ruin a human being. The waste that is so much of work of course makes people sad. How can this truth not count as we think about our mental health? When the basic mechanics of survival tax us, how can they not be factored in? All a mental health professional need ask is, "How's work going?" If the person across from her says, "Great!" and means it, she can sigh a huge sigh of relief. But if he says, "Oh, you know, it's just a paycheck," then the extravagant distress caused by being forced to earn a living doing meaningless work must be put on the table.

What follows on the heels of all of this distress—and I've named only two of the possible dozens of sources of that distress: the conflict between values and self-interest and the indignity of meaningless work—are completely predictable efforts at soothing ourselves and reducing the pain. Billions drink and use drugs. Billions join religions where soothing promises are made. Billions amuse themselves, invest time and energy in their sports teams, buy shoes, search out pornography, read romances, eat around the clock, create drama, or rail at their children. To reel from distress and rabidly root for your team or read two romances a day, these are not diseases. It is what we do to reduce our experience of distress. If we honored the reality of all that distress, we might become much slower to label.

Currently we are not giving distress its due. Consider someone you might expect to have some decent awareness of the realities of distress: Sigmund Freud. It so distressed Freud to have anyone disagree with his views that he broke off every friendship at the first whiff of disagreement. To soothe himself in the face of distress, he smoked cigars and couldn't stop smoking them even after he was diagnosed with mouth cancer. The father of psychoanalysis handled his distress no better than the next person. Whether we should pity him or shake our heads or wag a finger, if we mean to help ourselves, we had better not leave the centrality of distress—and our difficulties in dealing with distress—out of our equations.

We would be more inclined to pay this distress its due and more inclined to train our mental service providers to address it if people wore their distress on their sleeve. As it is, personality weaves itself around distress. We do not see the irritant that makes the pearl; more often than not, we can't see the distress around which this odd, sad, anxious, or critical personality has organized itself. Let me give you an example. Consider a client of mine I'll call John. I was doing a first coaching session with John via Skype. Because we both had our cameras on, I could see his environment. It was a shambles. So, too, was John. If you were a director and wanted to cast John, you would say to your casting director, "I need someone overweight, a loner, someone weird but not flat-out crazy." Your casting director would nod. We can all picture John.

John is difficult. When John tells me that his wife has recently divorced him, internally I think, "Yes, of course," and, "Wow, someone married you?" John claims not to be happy, partly because there is something missing in his life (he calls it "meaning"), partly because he is not suited to life (he feels that he is too quick and too smart), and partly because of external circumstances, namely that no business sees his worth and is willing to hire him on as a consultant. To someone observing him, his problems seem different. He seems awkward, immature, lacking in insight, unlovable, incapable of following through on much of anything. You palpably feel that "something is wrong with him" and that "something happened to him." He seems disturbed.

We look at him and in the absence of knowing what is really going on—and in large measure because he is so unhelpful, so difficult, so unaware, so talkative, so self-absorbed, and so out of touch with reality—we feel compelled to label John and throw in the towel. Distress must be at the root of all this. But John's grandiose style so puts us off that we find little room in our mind or our heart to look for the irritants that produced this human being. Whether we want to conceive of John as biologically broken, psychologically broken, strained but not broken, or in some other light, in the absence of knowing what is going on, it still remains our duty to remember that he is built to experience distress. But how hard he makes it for a helper to help him!

We are seduced into not understanding the evolutionary naturalness of distress for two reasons. First, when we feel this distress, we are inclined to believe that we have been visited by it, that "something" has happened out of the ordinary, something almost occult, as if some enemy has breathed this anxiety or sadness into us. We want to disown the distress, just as we want to disown diabetes or cancer. If the experience of sadness is like the experience of wearing a heavy overcoat, it is natural that we picture ourselves shedding it. This inclination to believe that we would be perfectly fine except for the visitation of this outside thing causes us to create two pictures of ourselves: an everyday well self and a burdened, visited self. Just like that we get it into our heads that we "have" something or have "caught" something.

This seduction is maintained by our desire to not take responsibility, not make changes, not control what we can control or influence what we can influence, not look too closely in the mirror, and not adopt the attitude that life purpose, meaning, and mental health are our projects. We avoid accepting our role in the situation. We stand surprisingly ready to abdicate our life in the face of the hardness of living. This ready abdication leads us to a willingness to accept one or another current mental disorder label because "having a mental disorder" is neither our fault nor our responsibility, and we are spared the shame and disappointment of having contributed to our own malaise.

The second reason we are seduced into not understanding the evolutionary naturalness of distress is that when we see someone with a disheveled personality, or someone manically racing through life, we have the sure sense that they are "off" in some way that a creature expressing its genes correctly could never be. We feel keenly that they have been visited by something that has ruined them. Was it their mother (a possibility that gives rise to psychotherapy)? Was it their brain chemistry (a possibility that gives rise to psychiatry)? That's how we all think. We look at someone who looks broken and believe that they could not be this way unless something is broken inside them. We find it hard to believe that they may simply be responding to distress in a particular way and that "broken" may not be the appropriate metaphor.

It would be nice if human beings could be given a head start and were taught that all this distress is coming. We could do this in our schools in addition to teaching history, math, and language skills. Right now, school is constructed to fill up our youth with information, socialize them, keep them off the streets, and allow their parents to work. School is not constructed to help our species deal with its evolutionary nature. For our general mental health to improve, a spectacular starting point would be helping our children enter into a new relationship with the distress they currently experience and are bound to experience in the future.

We could teach them to appreciate the naturalness and inevitability of distress and we could provide them with tactics for reducing and relieving their distress. These two skill sets can be taught and learned. Children can be taught that it is natural for them to distress over a lack of love, a lack of safety, a lack of predictability, and other everyday horrors. They can also be taught methods to help prevent them from organizing their personality around unaddressed irritants. Every school could have a human experience specialist of the sort I'll describe later whose express job would be to help children understand human nature, deal with their humanity, and prepare for the inevitable arrival of distress.

Let's return to John for a moment. He is grandiose and disheveled. But why isn't that his right? Why are these characteristics markers of a disorder or proof that he is broken? We experience John as disagreeable, difficult, uncooperative, and antisocial. But so what? Why can't John be that way? Well, you might say, he is obviously "impaired." But if that only means that he isn't doing the things we would like him to do or that we think are in his best interests, what right do we have to label him with a "mental disorder"? Well, it comes down to this feeling we can't shake that he just must be broken. He just must be. But is he?

Distress is a result. We hate our job and distress mounts. But distress is also a cause. We are distressed because we hate our job, and as the distress mounts, we have trouble sleeping, lose our appetite, or find little pleasure in our pastimes and pursuits. Thus we arrive at the things nowadays called "symptoms of depression." Life causes distress and distress then causes "symptoms." The mental health profession has lost its way and has chosen to focus on the symptoms and not the distress. When someone arrives in great distress, we are pulled to "identify symptoms" and label rather than inquire in part because human beings are difficult and tricky. It is much easier to prescribe a pill than deal with a person. There is little place to talk about distress as cause or distress as result. We are not much inclined to talk about that thousand-pound weight crushing your back.

Were we to return our focus to first causes—one being the reality of distress—we would instantly improve our mental health services.

At this point in the history of mental health theory and practice, we do not know if a person who presents with something we currently call a "mental disorder" or a "mental disease" should be considered "broken" or "not broken." We don't know what the realities are and we don't know what the right metaphors are. We can't say where John came from or what is really up with him. We can't articulate what his "problem" is or even if he has a problem. Nor should we call him disordered just because we think he must be. His appearance, his surroundings, his style, and his utterances all make us want to pin a label on him. We must refrain from doing that for reasons I'll explain shortly, and we must presume that distress is present. It is present in every life, and it must be present in John's, too.

Currently we do not possess a sensible or workable definition of mental disorder. We've been fooled into relying on so-called symptoms and symptom pictures as the way to "diagnose and treat mental disorders." We've come to call chemicals with powerful effects medication even though there is no clear indication that any disease or disorder is present. We've left the person out of the equation and we make patients out of people simply because they enter a certain sort of office where in fact nothing genuinely medical is taking place. We make zero distinctions between what is psychological and what is biological. We claim that an unwanted distressing thought or feeling is a sign of a disorder as opposed to simply being an unwanted distressing thought or feeling. There is much that we need to rethink and undo. One place of welcome housecleaning would be to sweep away the idea that human distress is an unnatural thing. It is as natural as breathing.

3

Jettisoning Normal

Our second piece of housecleaning is to brush "normal" and "abnormal" right out the door.

Normal and abnormal are not words like sweet and sour, green and red, or brick and mortar. Normal and abnormal are opinion words with multiple meanings and countless usages that are typically and regularly employed to persuade and manipulate. It is mind-boggling that the mental health industry is built on these two words that are about as solid as sand.

You may presume that the mental health establishment makes some wise, coherent distinctions between normal and abnormal. They do not. This is another place where you had better be skeptical of the putative expertise of so-called experts. It is past the time for us to abandon the words "normal" and "abnormal" as they pertain to the mental states and behaviors of human beings. It is a real question whether these words can be reasonably used at all, given their baggage, built-in biases, and the general confusion they create.

Is it really important that we look at the usage of these two words? It is. This isn't an idle question without real-world consequences. The "treatment" of every single "mental disorder" that mental health professionals "diagnose," from "depression" and "attention deficit disorder" on through "schizophrenia," flows from the way society allows its expert to construe "normal" and "abnormal." This matter affects tens of millions of people annually; it affects everyone, really, since who nowadays isn't flirting with a "mental disorder"?

What do you think "normal" and "abnormal" mean?

The matter of what is normal can't be and must not be a mere statistical nicety. It can't be and must not be "normal" to be a Christian just because 95 percent of your community is Christian. It can't be and must not be "normal" to be attracted to someone of the opposite sex just because 90 percent of the general population is heterosexual. It can't be and must not be "normal" to own slaves just because all the landowners in your state own slaves. "Normal" can't mean and must not mean "what we see all the time" or "what we see the most of." It must have a different meaning for it to mean anything of value to right-thinking people.

Nor can it mean "free of discomfort," as if "normal" were the equivalent of oblivious and you are somehow "abnormal" when you are sentient, human, and real. This, however, is the game currently being played by the mental health industry: it makes this precise, illegitimate switch. It announces that when you feel a certain level of discomfort, you are abnormal and have a disorder. It equates abnormal with unwanted, turning "I am feeling profoundly sad" into "You have the mental disorder of depression."

In this view, "normal" is living free of excessive discomfort; "abnormal" is feeling or acting significantly distressed. Normal, in this view, is destroying a village in wartime and not experiencing anything afterward; abnormal is experiencing something afterward and for a long time thereafter. The consequences of conscience, reason, and awareness are labeled abnormal, and robotic allegiance to wearing a pasted-on smiley face is designated normal. Is that what we really mean? Is that what you want "normal" and "abnormal" to mean?

Sadness, guilt, rage, disappointment, confusion, doubt, anxiety, and other similar experiences and states are all expected and normal, given the nature and demands of life; except, that is, to mental health professionals, where those states and experiences become markers of abnormality and cash cows. It is simply not right to call the absence of significant distress normal and the presence of significant distress abnormal. Does that seem right to you?

If "normal" mustn't be "what we see the most of" or "the absence of significant distress," how else might it be conceptualized or construed? Is there perhaps a way that the words "healthy" and "unhealthy" capture what we would like words such as "normal" and "abnormal" to mean? Perhaps "normal" could equal "healthy" and "abnormal" could equal "unhealthy"? Unfortunately, that emperor is also naked.

It is reasonable to say that if you contract tuberculosis or manifest cancer, you have gone from a healthier state to an unhealthier state. But it is not reasonable to say, for instance, that it is "healthy" to suffer no ill effects from killing unarmed civilians and "unhealthy" to experience distressing consequences. Yes, in the latter case you are suffering, but PTSD in this instance is not like cancer. In fact, it may amount to the healthy (and nevertheless extremely distressing) functioning of your conscience. This PTSD may be proof that you are healthy, proof, that is, that you are a person with a functioning conscience, rather than proof of any "unhealthiness."

It is not legitimate to announce that a person is "healthy" because she is not feeling distressed and "unhealthy" because she is feeling distressed. Growing sad because you caught your mate cheating on you doesn't make you "unhealthy." Growing anxious because you can't pay your bills doesn't make you "unhealthy." Growing bored and restless because your job underutilizes you doesn't make you "unhealthy." If you leap from "I am distressed" to "I am unhealthy," you are dangerously leaping into the arms of the pseudo-medical model.

The Twenty-Nine Senses of Normal

The mental disorder business, where folks sit around a table and turn "symptom pictures" into "mental disorders," rests on the Orwellian conceit that the average person is gullible enough to believe that there is a clear meaning to the word "normal" and a clear meaning to the word "abnormal." Anyone able to give the matter a second's thought will see that these words have so many usages as to empty them of meaning. (And if you don't agree with me, you're not normal!)

Here, to make the matter more explicit, are twenty-nine ways that the word "normal" is regularly used:

1. Normal = customary
   It is normal for a human being to believe in gods.
2. Normal = customary in context
   It was normal for French postmodernists to wear kimonos and other unusual attire.
3. Normal = predictable
   Given that he was hungry, that no one was watching, and that the apple pie was just sitting there, it was normal for him to steal a piece.
4. Normal = desirable
   It isn't normal for our kids not to want their own kids.
5. Normal = acceptable
   It isn't normal for a person to walk out during the eulogy. People should know better.
6. Normal = time limited
   It was normal for her to feel sad about the death of her husband, but it's been two years now.
7. Normal = possible
   Since some human beings have been cannibals, eating your enemy is a normal human behavior.

8. Normal = motivated
Once we understood her motives, her behavior struck us as completely normal.

9. Normal = rational
He answered all of my questions in a completely rational manner and seemed normal to me.

10. Normal = happy
She'd been unhappy for a long time, but she's more normal now, more like her old self.

11. Normal = becalmed
He'd been anxious for months before the premiere of his play, but he's much more normal now.

12. Normal = free of torment
I had no idea he was so tormented by crazy existential angst about the meaning of life! I thought he was more normal than that.

13. Normal = restrained
He used to flare up terribly and get enraged, but he's much more normal now.

14. Normal = controlled
Johnny used to be so fidgety in class, but now that he's on those three medications, he can sit still like a normal student.

15. Normal = self-interested
It is completely normal to not want to blow the whistle at work if that would cost you your job.

16. Normal = not sad
He was feeling blue at his last job, but he's feeling much more normal at his new job.

17. Normal = average
His intelligence falls within the normal range.

18. Normal = moral
Adulterers are sinners. They aren't normal.

19. Normal = legal or nearly legal
It's normal to drive a little over the speed limit, but he was going ninety.

20. Normal = age appropriate
That's normal behavior for a two year old.

21. Normal = developmentally appropriate
It's normal to act and feel that way when you leave home for the first time.

22. Normal = free of compulsion
He used be an alcoholic, but now he can drink normally.

23. Normal = free of obsession
He used to obsess about meeting Marilyn Monroe in Heaven, but now he has normal thoughts.

24. Normal = free of biological defect
His brain tumor is preventing him from thinking and acting normally.

25. Normal = free of psychological defect
How could anyone be normal with a mother like that?

26. Normal = free of spiritual defect
    The devil got hold of him for a few years, but he fought the devil off and is normal again.
27. Normal = free of personality defects
    Her shyness was really hampering her, but now she can speak up like a normal person.
28. Normal = free of social defect
    He was living a very isolated life, but now he goes out like any normal person.
29. Normal = free of some unnamable defect
    We can't say what's wrong with him, but he just isn't normal.

Have I captured every sense and usage of the word "normal"? Of course I haven't. Are some of these innocent enough and hardly worth railing against? Naturally. But the main point remains. The word "normal" is too slippery to be saved.

Is a cannibal normal? Is a kimono-clad postmodernist normal? Is a widow still grieving normal? Is a passive, medicated child normal? Is it more normal to drink or more normal to abstain? Everything can be normal when turned this way or that! And, dangerously, everything is abnormal. When we use words this loosely, they become weapons.

More than a hundred years of language analysis still hasn't helped us realize that the words we use matter. It is perhaps not in the nature of our species—not normal (wink, wink)—for a sufficient number of people to care enough about the terrible consequences of lame naming, consequences like forcing three, four, or five "normalizing" medications on a child. But we ought to care, because until we shed that unfortunate language, we can't think very clearly about cause and effect in human affairs. And the subtleties of cause and effect ought to interest us!

Consider the following. Imagine five young boys growing up in the same group home where they are repeatedly and severely beaten. One grows up to be a ruthless businessman who makes a fortune. A second grows up to be a serial killer. A third grows up to be a repressed priest with a penchant for visiting discipline-and-bondage porn sites. A fourth grows up to be a loving family man afflicted with bad memories, stomach problems, and difficulty concentrating. A fifth becomes a tortured poet who writes gorgeous, heart-felt poetry about pain and suffering who kills himself when he is twenty-eight.

Which of these are "normal" people and which are "abnormal" people? Which of these are "normal" outcomes and which of these are "abnormal" outcomes? Do those words help us at all or do they only get in the way of what we know to be true: that very different outcomes can arise from similar causes? Through a glass darkly, we see cause and effect at work here. The fingerprints of that seminal experience of brutality can be seen all over each outcome. We may despair about all of these outcomes: but that is not the same as saying that any one of them is "normal" or "abnormal." It is not like one of these five boys broke his arm and the other four didn't. All got broken. These outcomes make human sense.

A New Normal

What might a "new normal" look like? We would never call it that, as we really do mean to expunge the words "normal" and "abnormal." But let's be light-hearted about it for a moment and try our hand at painting a beginning picture of a "new normal."

When you fall from a tree and break your arm, we say that you injured your arm. We do not call you abnormal. Can't we be that simple, sensible, and real in regard to sadness, psychological pain, overwhelm, anxiety, inner turmoil, and the other commonly occurring and understandable psychological events that members of our species face? Can't we stop calling them "symptoms of disease" and calling ourselves "abnormal" for experiencing them?

Isn't it time that we break free of the mesmerizing forces that want us to avoid looking the reality of our human condition in the eye? If we could do that, if we could adopt a "new normal" that let quintessential human experiences into our definition of normal, we could begin to create a way of speaking and practical strategies, tactics, and plans that return the tasks of living to those embroiled in it.

"Normal" would now include pain, difficulty, and struggle. We would possess a "new normal" that caught up with our understanding of who we are and how we got here. If you believe that our species has evolved and was not created out of whole cloth, you should likewise realize that normal mental health aligns much more with the idea of struggle than with the idea of tranquility. We have evolved as a creature with roiling insides. To leave all that roiling, all that turmoil, all that sadness and pain out of our definition of normal mental health is to make a fundamental error.

Why does a child sit as his desk as his teacher lectures? He sits there with his hands folded because he is coerced and socialized, not because he has any desire to be there. What is normal for him and what his being wants is to have him leap up and run off to play. What is normal for him are his squirming, his making faces, and his expression of outrage at being forced to learn a list of Roman emperors or Spanish missions of California. He is struggling to sit there, not happy to sit there. If we do not honor that struggle as a feature of normal mental health, we make a mockery out of the word "normal."

A person may write one novel after another because she has ideas for novels, loves novels, and experiences writing novels as a place of meaning. At the same time, no one may publish her novels or, if she decides to self-publish them, buy them or read them. This is a completely normal outcome in the world of creativity and the world of competition, a typical struggle, and it is likely to produce great frustration, inner turmoil, and sadness. In what universe can it be abnormal to experience frustration, inner turmoil, and sadness at having no one take an interest in your creations?

It is a bad joke to tell people that it is abnormal to mourn the loss of a son long dead, abnormal to feel squeamish flying through a hurricane, abnormal to rage against a rapist to the point of hating the universe itself, abnormal to cry out in disgust at watching a marathon of a favorite sitcom, abnormal to eat every brownie in the house when appetite rages inside, abnormal to career from one mood to another. None of this is abnormal.

Our current normal is of great use to anyone who is paid to see us as afflicted as opposed to human. True normal, by contrast, is an hour of peace, a minute of rage, fifteen minutes of frustration, a week of meaninglessness, a day of love, a year of confusion, an hour of awe, an entire life of helpless awareness coupled with acute distress, and our effective and ineffective efforts at relief. That is true normal!

If this new normal were our currency, a person would be able to say, "It is completely normal that I am in great psychological pain because of my miserable marriage; my dull, stressful job; and my abiding feeling that life is a cheat. This emotional pain is normal given my life and my belief system. But it is not okay with me! Here is what I am going to do to minimize my pain. I am getting a divorce. I am getting into a new line of work. I am changing my mind about life. I am going to do a lot! Because the pain, while completely normal, is not acceptable to me!"

With this upgraded view of normal, you could construct your emotional health your way. You could say, "Life is a struggle, pain is coming, and here are my intentions." You could say, "Forget about some crazy notion of tranquility! Forget about tranquilizers. Here is my plan for meeting this great struggle." We would begin to self-define emotional health in terms not of happiness but of our relationship to struggle.

Taking this evolutionary view we would begin to include a wide range of experiences, the terrible and the poignant together, in our definition of normal. Finally we could spend real time, the most valuable time we could possibly spend, painting a picture for ourselves of what constitutes bearable living. We could begin to focus on distress reduction, pain relief, tactics for coping with struggle, and ways to invite in occasional happiness. You don't tell an antelope, "With this drug you will be cured of tigers." You shouldn't tell a person, "With this drug you will be cured of struggle." Rather you should say, "Struggle is the preeminent feature of nature." Our new normal would include this reality. With it we could paint a beautiful picture, beautiful because of its honesty, of our exquisite acceptance of the realities of human pain and struggle, and the creation of wise tactics for dealing with that pain and struggle.

Upgrading Normal

Our "new normal" would include the truth that people face difficulties. But it must also include the truth that people are themselves difficult. Let's take a look at a few thumbnail sketches of modern life to drive this point home.

Two educated people who do not particularly want a child have one. The father works a lot and isn't interested in the baby. The mother, unfulfilled and herself uninterested in the baby, adopts the persona of super-mom, as she doesn't know what else to do with herself. She watches the little boy and measures him every moment. Is he crawling fast enough? Is he adept enough at his little computer? Are his fingers long enough to play the piano at a concert level? Can he keep up with the other kids at story time? Since he appears to be behind in all of these regards, she gets him help: drugs to help his fingers grow, tutors to press him on his computer skills, and a story-time specialist to help him sing along better.

At three, still behind but now irritable, withdrawn, and on the brink of not being Stanford or Harvard material, and, maybe worse, not getting into the best preschool, he is brought to the big-gun experts where he gets his ADHD, childhood depression, and other labels, each of which comes with a chemical solution and an accommodation. This is one version of our modern parent and our modern child.

How can we talk about the "mental health" of this three-year-old without concerning ourselves with the personalities and motives of his parents and his putative helpers?

A cruel, abusive, heavy-drinking father and his passive, church-going, half-invalid wife do not notice that their daughter is frightened and miserable. What they do notice is that she loves dancing, which angers the father, as he hates anyone enjoying anything, and likewise infuriates the mother, who underneath her passivity is exactly as furious and mean-spirited as her husband. The father yells and the mother flings Biblical passages. When it can't help but be noticed at school that this young girl is concentration camp thin, everyone agrees that she has an eating disorder. As her mother puts it, "She's always been stubborn."

How can we talk about the "mental health" of this rail-thin girl without taking into account the difficult people on all sides of her against whom she is defending herself?

A privileged youth drops out of college to "find himself." Because his parents will not pay for his proposed five-year exploration of world poetry, and because work would prove too taxing and boring, he becomes fat. He also becomes a minister. His "poetic quest" becomes a "spiritual quest." As soon as he is ordained, he decides that the job of minister is too mundane for him, plus his disabilities prevent him from getting anywhere on time, taking orders, listening, or functioning even slightly in the workaday world. So, by talking fast and by issuing threats, he manages to parlay his ADHD, his bipolar disorder, and his other mental disorders into a "complete disability" diagnosis, a nice tax-free monthly check, and the opportunity to eat a lot and read French poetry. He has just about every mental disorder a person can have—and yet, lo and behold, he doesn't seem particularly unhappy.

How can we talk about his "mental health" without factoring in human willfulness?

A gay actor who has lived with his gay lover for a decade is asked by his publicist to participate in a documentary about "his great love affair with Adrienne." "Who's Adrienne?" he asks. "Doesn't matter," she replies. "We'll cast someone." He agrees, knowing that he has to appear straight in order to work in Hollywood. The documentary is made and his publicist books him on all the morning talk shows, all the midday talk shows, and all the late night talk shows. His female fans can hardly wait to hear about his great love affair! At the last minute, his appearances have to be cancelled because he's "had a nervous breakdown" and has signed himself into a deluxe desert resort rest home. When asked what he's suffering from, his publicist replies, "Food poisoning." Soon the actor is able to ink a multi-million dollar deal to play a macho cartoon action hero.

How can we talk about the "mental health" of this gay actor without acknowledging the games that people knowingly play—games with predictable emotional consequences that, however, the players involved never seem to expect?

It isn't just that "normal" and "abnormal" are pliable words with multiple meanings and contradictory usages. It's that what passes for normal in human affairs is shockingly inadequate. "Normal" isn't a rock upon which to build an edifice. It is a quagmire from which we must extricate ourselves. We need to improve "normal." Part of our agenda for the future of mental health is painting a picture of how low we have set the bar, where we might want to set it, and how we can help people upgrade themselves.

Our new human experience specialist would see that as a significant part of the job. Our specialists would tell the parents of that three-year-old, "Maybe loving him would help." They would tell the parents of that rail-thin girl, "Can't you see she's miserable?" They would tell that bloated ex-minister, "You talk a good game." They would tell that gay actor, "Really? You expected to participate in this charade and not get a little sick to your stomach?" Might customers walk out? Indeed they might, as the truth is rarely well received. Still, telling the truth comes right at the top of the job description.

In each of the above scenarios, there are mental health establishment players ready, willing, and able to provide diagnoses and offer up treatment options. Happy to diagnose that three-year-old! Happy to diagnose that miserable girl! Happy to diagnose that stay-at-home minister! Happy to diagnose that closeted actor! Not to worry—we pledge not to look at what's going on. Never fear—we will hold no one responsible. Our new human experience specialist, however, will not play along. Using whatever skill and tact they can muster to have a chance of being heard, our specialists will point a sharp finger.

She rejects the words "normal" and "abnormal" because they signify too little, carry too much baggage, and let people off the hook. She knows that "normal" and "abnormal" are not innocent words. They are loaded words regularly used against you by the mental health establishment. By virtue of the fact that they can mean just about anything, the mental health establishment has taken them to mean certain insupportable things. We have to call that establishment on their usage.

At the same time, she knows that what passes for "normal" among human beings is a level of functioning and a level of human decency far below what we might want it to be. It is "normal" for people to experience difficulties, but it is also "normal" for people to handle their difficulties poorly and to turn into difficult and sometimes dangerous creatures. We want to get rid of the words "normal" and "abnormal" and substitute much more sensible, intelligible terms.

4

Rethinking Diagnosis

Imagine that you got upset. Is it very remarkable that I can "diagnose" that you are upset? After all, you are clearly upset. What expert thing did I accomplish by agreeing with you that you were upset?

Imagine that you are angry. Is it very remarkable that I can "diagnose" that you are angry? After all, you are clearly angry. Have I added anything meaningful by saying "I diagnose that you are angry" instead of "You seem angry"?

"You look upset" is the simple, truthful thing to say, and "I diagnose that you look upset" is a piece of self-serving chicanery. By adopting that circumlocution, I've tried to turn an ordinary observation into a pseudo-scientific marvel. If this is the way I'm operating, I dearly hope that you won't notice my little game.

By contrast, let's say that you explain to me that you've been having hallucinations. You describe the look of your hallucination, and you also describe to me your recent history, other physical symptoms, and so on. Taking that information together, I have a strong hunch that you're suffering from early Parkinson's. I then run tests to confirm or disconfirm my hypothesis. I didn't "diagnose" your hallucination—you handed me that. I diagnosed your Parkinson's.

We seem to have a lot of trouble understanding this difference: the difference between "diagnosing a symptom" and "diagnosing a cause." The second is what medicine legitimately does. The first is what the mental health establishment illegitimately does. It is not real diagnosis for me to "diagnose you with an anxiety disorder" because you told me you were anxious. This is chicanery and not diagnosis.

You don't diagnose symptoms. You diagnose causes. To diagnose a symptom is only to say, "Yes, I agree, you have a rash." Everyone who looks at you knows that you have a rash! What we want to know is what sort of rash it is. What's causing it? You observe the tumor and diagnose the cancer. You observe the bump and diagnose the concussion. You observe the fever and diagnose the influenza. You don't observe the anxiety and diagnose the anxiety. That is wrong.

You observe a symptom, you interpret a symptom, and you make use of a symptom as part of your efforts at diagnosis. But the symptom isn't the diagnosis. You observe a symptom and then diagnose a cause. You don't observe anxiety and then diagnose anxiety. It isn't okay to call this "diagnosing." It isn't okay to turn a report of anxiety into "an anxiety disorder" just by saying so. Yet this is what is done all the time nowadays.

Here, for example, are some of the questions whose positive answer will get you an "anxiety disorder" diagnosis:

- "Are you feeling keyed up or on edge?"
- "Do you have feelings of panic, fear, or uneasiness?"
- "Are you constantly worrying about small or large concerns?"
- "Are you constantly tense?"
- "Does your anxiety interfere with your work, school, or family responsibilities?"
- "Are you plagued by fears that you know are irrational, but can't shake?"
- "Do you avoid everyday situations or activities because they cause you anxiety?"
- "Do you watch for signs of danger?"

If you answer yes to these questions, you are acknowledging in these different-but-same ways that you are feeling anxious. But what you get from the mental health establishment is not, "Yes, you are clearly feeling anxious. Let's see if we can figure out why." What you get is a "diagnosis" of an "anxiety disorder." In our current system, you appear to have "symptoms" of an "anxiety disorder." You come in looking anxious, acting anxious, and saying that you are anxious. What sort of diagnostic acumen does it take for me to say, "You're anxious"?

Let's look at a hypothetical fellow. Jim has looked a certain way his whole life: he has been recognizably himself for as long as he or anyone can remember. If you are his mate or his friend, you are pretty much certain how he'll react if, say, you offer him a second beer, ask him if he wants to climb a mountain, ask him to play a board game, and so on. You know his likes and dislikes, his habits, his characteristic expressions, pretty much everything.

Jim goes away for a week and comes back different. This is a classic plot in fiction, where a character goes off for many years, say to war, and when he comes back his wife is certain that he isn't the same man but an impostor, even though he looks the same, has all the right memories and information, and can pass any test on being himself. However, his wife just knows that he isn't the same man. Let's say that Jim, who has never seemed particularly anxious previously, comes home highly anxious.

He looks anxious. He says he's anxious. His anxiety is keeping him from sleeping. The question isn't, "Is Jim anxious?" The question is, "Why is Jim suddenly anxious, so much so that he doesn't even seem to be the same person?" To "diagnose" Jim with "an anxiety disorder" is child's play: he is clearly anxious. That is no diagnosis at all. That's like diagnosing Jim with "lump-itis" if he comes in with a baseball-sized lump on the side of his head. "Lump-itis" won't do. Nor will "anxiety disorder."

We want to know three things: Why is Jim anxious? What might we suggest to help Jim, given the particular source of his anxiety? And what can we suggest to help Jim whether or not we're able to discern why he is anxious? Too many mental health providers skip the first two questions because Jim may not cooperate in their investigation, because those "causes" are too hard to discern, and/or because those "causes" are frankly unknowable. They go directly to the third. They say, "Let's treat that anxiety!" They say, "Let's treat that symptom!" The pills appear; talk of a certain sort commences. No real investigation of the cause begins because steps one and two are assiduously skipped.

Jim's Week

Let's imagine that the following ten things occurred in Jim's life during the week that he was away:

1. On the flight home, his plane encountered engine trouble and had to be diverted to Amarillo.
2. He started an affair with a woman half his age and half his wife's age, an affair that he would like to continue even though he feels guilty about betraying his wife.
3. He took certain street drugs for the first time.
4. He had a memory that he couldn't shake about a test that he failed miserably in fourth grade and how his teacher humiliated him when she handed out the test results.
5. He experienced certain physical symptoms, including heart palpitations and sudden sweats.
6. He received an email and learned that he was about to be audited.
7. He had a nightmare in which he saw himself being drawn and quartered for his unpopular beliefs.
8. He received an email from his sister saying that she was unwilling to continue taking complete responsibility for caring for their demented mother.

9. He began wondering if misplacing his hotel key and his car keys were signs of his own early dementia.
10. He reread a portion of a novel he had once written, discovered that he still liked it, and began to wonder if he should resume writing it.

Whether or not any of these "caused" Jim's sudden anxiety, doesn't each feel suggestive and something like a potential clue? Wouldn't you want to know these things if you were tasked with helping Jim reduce his experience of anxiety? Forgetting for a second about how you might actually discern which of these, if any, was causing Jim's sudden onset of anxiety, don't we suspect that even just getting them named and "on the table" might have some salubrious effect on Jim? Doesn't all therapy that isn't caught up in "diagnosing and treating mental disorders" rely on this central idea, that making the unknown known helps people reduce their experience of distress?

We'd certainly like to possess that information about Jim's week. Let's add another wrinkle. What if Jim reports that he believes that the anxiety is the result of him being followed all week by a certain suspicious stranger—a man Jim is sure was there but who in fact wasn't. In this scenario, Jim may be suffering from an actual organic syndrome—and a feature of this organic syndrome may be that Jim will not believe you when you try to explain to him, if you are in a position to do so, that the stranger does not exist and could not have existed.

For example, patients with Anton's syndrome, which can arise in blind individuals with cortical damage, may "see" exactly such strangers as Jim feels he is seeing—and they can't be convinced that they are hallucinating. Oliver Sachs explained in *Hallucinations*, "A patient with Anton's syndrome, if asked, will describe a stranger in the room by providing a fluent and confident, though entirely incorrect, description. No argument, no evidence, no appeal to reason or common sense is of the slightest use."

This possibility should further highlight what investigating looks like. You can't learn this vital information if the transaction plays itself out in the following way, as it almost certainly will between Jim and a chemical-oriented psychiatrist:

"So, Jim, you're generally anxious?" says the psychiatrist, looking at the intake form.

"I am!"

"That means you have generalized anxiety disorder."

"Okay!"

"As it happens, I have some yellow pills, orange pills, and blue pills to treat that disorder. Let me tell you about them."

"Can't wait to hear!"

It should be perfectly clear that "diagnosing the symptom" ("You've got anxiety!") and then "treating the symptom" ("Here's a pill!") is simply the path of least resistance. We can see why it is so tempting to engage in this shortcut and this illegitimate process since it appears well nigh impossible to know whether Jim is anxious because his anxious nature, dormant "forever," suddenly kicked in; whether a single idle memory, say of that fourth grade humiliation, caused "all this emotional fuss"; whether the affair, the audit, or the near plane crash provoked this new anxiety; and so on. Rather than admit that he doesn't know what is causing the anxiety, probably can't know, and doesn't really care one way or the other, a chemical-oriented psychiatrist simply proceeds to "diagnose and treat the symptom."

We understand the temptation. There are no tests to connect these possible "causes" in any direct or indirect way to Jim's sudden onslaught of anxiety. For the most part, we simply can't know. Nor can Jim, for that matter. Maybe he reads over his list and exclaims, "It's the audit! That's what's doing it!" Do we trust Jim's judgment on this score? Do we believe that Jim is accurately ascribing the right cause from among all these plausible causes? Do we believe that a certain feeling, insight, or self-report on Jim's part amounts to an "accurate diagnosis" of the source of his anxiety?

Not if Jim is the tricky, complicated, evasive creature he surely is— namely, not if Jim is a human being. Can we really trust Jim, especially once we discover that he doesn't want to talk about how the new affair may be affecting him? Do we want to "diagnose" Jim with "audit-induced anxiety" because he's cherry picked the audit off his list? No. We know better than to take at face value the often self-serving explanations that human beings provide. We can't rely on Jim; we can't "test" Jim. And so, then what? Do we throw Jim to the chemical-oriented psychiatrist? No. Rather, we say to Jim, "You know, I wonder . . ."

This "wondering" might sound like the following:

"Jim, you've picked the audit as the main source of your anxiety. But what about the affair you're having and what about keeping that affair a secret from your wife? Isn't that likely implicated? Don't you think you might be suffering from a guilty conscience?"

"I don't feel guilty."

"But you said earlier that you did feel guilty."

"I do and I don't. The bottom line is, I don't want to end the affair, and I don't want my wife to know. I want to get rid of the anxiety, not end the affair."

"Oh. That is *so* interesting."

This is a perfectly clear, characteristic, and plausible exchange. Jim's part of the exchange can be translated as, "I want relief from the symptom, and I do not want to make any fundamental change in the way I'm operating. If you happen to have a pill handy, that would be lovely." Jim may well pull for that pill! And what frustrated helper wouldn't want to hand Jim the pill bottle and say, "Have it your way. This pill has strong effects that may quell your anxiety. I wash my hands of you and your nonsense. Let's collude in acting like the anxiety is a 'thing' that blew in through the open window and that we have 'medicine' for it. Fine. Let's play that game."

However, our human experience specialist, or any psychotherapist who doesn't feel obliged to "diagnose and treat symptom pictures," doesn't have to pull out the pill response. Our specialist can continue, one human being to another, "You want the affair, you want the lying, the hiding, the cheating, and all of that, and you don't want the anxiety that may come from the lying, the hiding, the cheating, and so on? Have I got that right? Tell me, Jim—does that make any sense to you?"

You investigate, you suggest, you hypothesize . . . and you tell the truth. There is a world of difference between "diagnosing and treating" and investigating, suggesting, hypothesizing, and telling the truth. When psychotherapists investigate, suggest, hypothesize, and tell the truth, they are helping; when they "diagnose the mental disorder of generalized anxiety disorder," they are playing a game, illegitimately labeling, and creating a pseudo-patient who, like Jim, may prefer to be a pseudo-patient than deal with the turn his life has taken. When they do the former, they deserve a well-earned round of applause; when they "diagnose," they ought not sleep well.

Consider the following. What if nothing unusual or provocative happened to Jim during his week away? Does that make Jim's anxiety uncaused? Of course it doesn't. It only means that we know even less about its source than if we had some obvious clues. In a certain sense that may even prove helpful, because without obvious clues, we can't leap to connecting up Jim's sudden anxiety with some too simple "cause." We would naturally presume that there are reasons for his heightened anxiety, reasons that we may never come to know, and even more adamantly invite Jim to collaborate in our investigation.

Let's say that Jim does collaborate and that he lands on that audit as the source of his anxiety. We may not completely believe him, but should we dispute him or ignore his formulation of the problem? No, we shouldn't. After we've said what we had to say, for example, about his affair, we might then want to take Jim at his word and consider the possibility that the upcoming audit is indeed the primary source of his anxiety. Given that Jim has said so, we might take that as a working hypothesis. A working hypothesis is very different from a diagnosis. When a doctor says, "It might be this, it might be this, it might be this, or it might be this," he is announcing his hypotheses. He hasn't made a diagnosis yet. Nor should we as we begin our investigations. In medicine, you don't diagnose until you can diagnose.

Will a moment come, in Jim's case or in any other, when we can "make a diagnosis"? I think the answer is a clear no. What could such a diagnosis sound like? Audit-induced anxiety reaction coupled with denial-induced extramarital affair-itis? Sudden Personality Change Syndrome caused by a plane's engine catching fire? Unleashed Primal Lust for Younger Woman Syndrome with overtones of guilt and pleasure? These human events can't and shouldn't be "diagnosed" as if they were illnesses. Let us stop looking to diagnosis as the Holy Grail. It isn't. Right now it is only a mechanism for turning human experience into mental health establishment profits.

Not Diagnosing at All

For the many professionals looking for decent alternatives to the current mental health labeling system and our methods of diagnosing, I would say that the best alternative to our current ways of diagnosing is to not diagnose at all. Let us understand diagnosing for what it is: an inappropriate lifting of a term and an idea from enterprises where it makes sense, like repairing cars and repairing hearts, to one where it doesn't. We will do much better as helpers without adding illegitimate "diagnosing" to our game plan.

A lawyer helps clients without diagnosing or labeling. An accountant helps clients without diagnosing or labeling. Our new human experience specialist can also help—as can any psychotherapist who rejects the pseudo-medical model—without diagnosing or labeling. If they are suffering from a medical illness, they should see a doctor, who has the job of diagnosing their Parkinson's or their Anton's syndrome. Diagnosing those real illnesses isn't the job of any psychotherapist on earth. Nor should it be their job to "diagnose" made-up ones.

The end of diagnosing doesn't imply the end of helping. It does imply the end of "treating," another medical word and idea. It would actually promote rather than impede helping. In a postdiagnosis future, you could say, "You're anxious. Let's investigate why because maybe that investigation will help us. And if we can't figure out why, that's okay too. We can still try out some things that may help you feel less anxious. And, who knows, they may even help with what's causing the anxiety. Okay? By the way, I will need your cooperation in this because I am not a doctor with tests and treatments and what-have-you. I am just a person like you. I'm willing to focus you a little, ask some pointed questions, be on your side when I feel I can be, and be 'in this' with you. But I need your help. Okay?"

This new human experience specialist would probably also have to say to Jim, "By the way, let's talk about pills for a second." That is, she would probably have to put on the table the fact that Jim can take certain chemicals-with-powerful-effects that might quell his anxiety. Maybe she'll have at her disposal a newly minted brochure sanctioned by the government that she could hand Jim that would spell out the "role of chemicals in altering human experience." At any rate, society might well demand that she have a pill chat with Jim and inform him of his right to take chemicals to deal with his anxiety. But let's leave the details of that difficult discussion aside for the moment.

To return to the main thread, can we help Jim even if we can't locate the "cause" of his anxiety? Can we legitimately decide to "treat" the "symptom" without identifying the "cause"? Of course we can. You can "treat a symptom" without "diagnosing a symptom." This happens all the time in medicine. You call your doctor late in the afternoon and say, "I have a headache." He says, "Take two aspirin and call me in the morning." He has not diagnosed you, but he is treating your symptom. History tells him that you will probably wake up without the headache for any one of three reasons: that the aspirin worked, that some placebo effect worked, or that the headache, like many headaches, just went away.

It is perfectly plausible, sensible, and reasonable to sometimes "just treat symptoms." We have plenty of things to recommend that might help a sad person, an anxious person, a person who drinks too much, and so on. Maybe a sad person would benefit from some sunlight, an anxious person from some "don't sweat the small stuff" training, a problem drinker from AA. But if the headaches persist, you don't just keep "treating the symptom"—you don't just keep recommending aspirins. You say to the person across from you, "Please, please, please, let's see if we can get at what's going on here. Okay? Can we please do a little investigating?"

In real life, you can do both: you can "treat the symptom" by providing some time-tested tactics, and you can also "investigate what's going on underneath." Indeed, this amounts to best practice. And nowhere in this best practice was there a need for diagnosing to rear its ugly head. Yet many well-meaning mental health professionals retain a desire to diagnose because they genuinely believe in the "diagnosing and treating" model. A well-known therapist dropped me the following note in response to a column of mine in *Psychology Today*:

I appreciate your position and understand your concern about using the word "diagnosis," but I think it is unfortunate that we have ceded this term entirely to medical practice. According to Merriam Webster's dictionary, diagnosis is the "investigation or analysis of the cause or nature of a condition, situation, or problem." By this definition, mental health disorder categories may not even qualify as diagnoses because by being "atheoretical" regarding cause, they offer little in terms of meaningful explanation that lends itself to helpful courses of action.

Psychological formulation, on the other hand, fits nicely with the idea of diagnosis as a process by which we come to identify and understand the problems clients present to their therapists. I'd go so far as to say that based on this definition, client and counselor could even diagnose a problem together—something quite different from the usual presumption that diagnosis is limited to the notion of expert therapists independently deciding what is wrong without client involvement. My point is that diagnosis need not be viewed in the very restricted sense it has been for so long in the helping professions.

I understand this desire, but this would still amount to a misuse of the word "diagnosis," and it would continue our current pattern of abusing both language and human beings. You discern causes, if you can; you don't co-create them. A human experience specialist and her client can certainly co-create a plan for managing anxiety, co-create an agreement about what the client will or won't try, and so on. All of that can be co-created. But you can't co-create a diagnosis. That's Monty Python territory.

The challenge for any contemporary psychotherapist who wants to retain an ability to "diagnose and treat" is simple to describe: give me an example of your updated diagnostic system. Tell me how you would test to confirm your diagnoses and how you would distinguish one cause or source of a problem from another cause or source of a problem. Give me your taxonomy—your naming system and your rationale for using it—and let's hold it up to scrutiny. If you want to continue diagnosing, put up the names of your "mental disorders" and let's look them over. And don't forget to clearly indicate what you are counting as causes! If you don't take causes into account, you still aren't really diagnosing. You are merely cataloguing.

I think that we will discover, if we are truthful and if we are acting in good faith, that it is impossible to retain the idea of "diagnosing" when it comes to human experiences. We should stop "diagnosing symptoms" right now, as that is a completely illegitimate enterprise that is annually adding millions of people, many of them children, to the rolls of the "mentally disordered." This should stop today. But we should also let go of the idea that "diagnosing and treating" makes any sense in the context of human experience. It is simple: we have adopted the wrong model. It is past time to discard it.

As to whether there is perhaps some way to retain the idea of "diagnosing," let those who want it retained describe what their taxonomy might look like and let us see if we believe them. I don't think we will believe them, because it is folly, and always will be folly, to "diagnose the human condition" when we have no way of knowing what counts as cause and effect in human affairs. Are we to "diagnose" personality differences, changed circumstances, stray and odd thoughts, and every single human thing, from war breaking out to a month of cloudy days? Such an enterprise makes no sense.

We do not know what caused Jim to become anxious, and while we can investigate his situation with him, we can't arrive at the sorts of conclusions that in medicine are called "diagnoses." To announce that we can arrive at such conclusions or that such conclusions are warranted by our investigations is to lie. We can help Jim a lot—and we will help Jim a lot more if we stop "diagnosing" him and simply start helping him. That should be our rallying cry: "Lots of help and no more diagnosing!"

A doctor is not engaged in idle investigating. He is trying to succeed in his investigations. We do not think that a doctor has been successful if he engages in one surgery after another to find out "what is wrong with us." In that unfortunate set of circumstances, he has not reached a conclusion yet, and so he can't make a diagnosis. If there ever was a way to "diagnose" in human affairs—and there never will be—we would need to set the bar exactly that high: we would need to be successful in our investigations, and we would need to be able to say, "This is clearly causing that." That time can never come.

A diagnosis is a conclusion about cause and effect. "You need new spark plugs" is a conclusion about cause and effect. "You say you are anxious, so I will say that you are anxious" is not a conclusion about cause and effect. It is time for society, in the form of its legislators and watchdogs, to end this travesty. Millions upon millions of adults and children are receiving "diagnoses" that make no earthly sense. And these "diagnoses" stay with them forever. Mention that you are sad to the wrong person and you will carry a "clinical depression" label with you everywhere.

It is time we placed a moratorium on this illegitimate "diagnosing." No new system will prove legitimate because we do not actually know what "causes" individual human experiences like sadness and anxiety. It is simply improper to turn human experiences, even of the most painful and unwanted sort, into "disorders." Let us help with the pain; let us really help Jim. And let us leave "diagnosing" to car mechanics and their faulty carburetors and to medical doctors and their Anton's syndromes.

5

What Shall We Call You?

You are in distress and seek help. Let's name certain kinds of distress to help us visualize who you are. Maybe you feel sad or "depressed." Maybe you feel even darker than that: maybe you're despairing or suicidal. Maybe you feel anxious. Maybe you believe that you're suffering from an addiction. Maybe your behaviors are out of control, and you've sought out help. Maybe someone else, maybe a parent or the courts, have demanded that you get help. Maybe your distress is of the sort that gets called "serious mental illness"—maybe, for example, you are delusional or "schizophrenic." Maybe you're having relationship problems, maybe you feel isolated and lonely. Maybe you feel under tremendous stress at work. Maybe you are having "trouble with life" and want a sympathetic ear and some new strategies and tactics for living.

You want help. But before we can discuss what help is available to you and, in particular, what our human experience specialist might have to offer you, we need to know what to call you. I hope I've convinced you that the naming of things is no innocent business. It matters if there really are "mental disorders" or if we are only designating certain thoughts, feelings, and behaviors as such. It matters if there is something sensible to say about "normal" and "abnormal" or if we are using those words inappropriately and primarily to make money. And—this is what we want to examine next—it matters if it is proper to call you a "patient" or if it isn't.

Why should someone experiencing emotional distress be labeled a "patient"? Shouldn't we reserve the word "patient" for genuine medical interactions? The current mental health system promotes the idea that mental health service providers "see patients." This ought to change. The practice is both illegitimate and dangerous. Why dangerous? First of all, "just like that" you have given me license to see you in a certain way: as sick. Patients are not sick people by definition, since you may see a doctor and learn that you are just fine. Yet the word "patient" carries with it the large likelihood that you are, in fact, sick. By accepting that label, you have accepted a certain sort of verdict, one that has not been adjudicated.

If you are a service provider, will you see me as "sick" just by virtue of the label I'm wearing? You quite likely will. Say, for example, that I'm a well-known mental health professional. I tell you, another mental health professional, that the "patient" I'm sending over to you, a person who is completely mentally healthy, "appears neurotic but is really psychotic." What are the chances that you will agree with my diagnosis in the absence of any actual evidence of "neurosis" or "psychosis"? According to one elegant experiment, 100 percent!

There looks to be a 100 percent chance that, even if I am well, you will see me as sick because a colleague of yours told you that I'm sick. In an experiment performed by Maurice Temerlin and reported in the *Journal of Nervous and Mental Disease*, Temerlin had an actor memorize a script designed to portray a mentally healthy individual whom we'll call Harry. Harry was happy, effective at work, self-confident, warm, gracious, happily married, and insightful—as mentally healthy as a person can be.

Harry's performance, presented as an "intake interview," was played for a group of mental health professionals. Beforehand, a well-known mental health professional told the gathered group that they were about to listen to an interview with a man who "appears neurotic but is really psychotic." After listening to Harry, they were told to rate Harry's mental health based only on the interview; they were explicitly told not to use the information provided by the "prestige associate."

The results? Virtually every graduate student, clinical psychologist, and psychiatrist rated Harry as either neurotic or psychotic. The psychiatrists were the worst in this regard: 60 percent rated him psychotic and 40 percent rated him neurotic. Having listened to an interview with a healthy man and having been told to confine their ratings to the evidence of that interview, 100 percent of the psychiatrists judged him disordered because a "prestige associate" told them that they ought to.

Multiple experiments have confirmed that when presented with a "patient" or a "prospective patient," mental health professionals are considerably more likely to "diagnose the presence of a mental disorder." The very act of walking in somehow confirms that you have a "mental disorder"! An excellent experiment run by Ellen Langer of Harvard and Robert Abelson of Yale and published in the *Journal of Consulting and Clinical Psychology* further illustrates this point.

The experimenters wanted to gauge what therapists would say about a subject who for one set of therapists was called a "job applicant" and who for a second set of therapists was called a "patient." Would the latter label bias their opinions? It did indeed. Therapists who thought that the subject was a job applicant used words like "candid," "upstanding," "innovative," and "ingenious" to describe him. Therapists who thought that the subject was a patient used words and phrases like "tight," "defensive," "frightened of his own aggressive impulses," "conflicted over homosexuality," and "passive dependent type" to describe him. The experimenters concluded, "Once an individual enters a therapist's office for consultation, he has labeled himself 'patient.' The therapist's negative expectations in turn may affect the patient's own view of the situation, thereby possibly locking the interaction into a self-fulfilling gloomy prophecy."

If there is a genuine illness present and it is a professional's job to treat illnesses, it is then fair to call folks "patients" when they walk into that professional's office. It is fair to call them "patients" even when they aren't suffering from an illness or disorder, just so long as the professional's office is truly a medical office and just so long as the professional can actually distinguish between health and illness. But what if the transaction is more of the following sort? Say that you enter a mental health service provider's office and share that you are worried about your son's drinking, the impending loss of your job, and your mate's infidelity, and that these pressures and many other pressures are making you unhappy. If, after I hear this, I say to you that you are "ill" with the "mental disorder of clinical depression," I have illegitimately labeled you and illegitimately turned you into a patient. You came in wanting to talk about your problems, and you left as a patient with a mental disorder.

Whether a professional's office carries the shingle of psychiatrist, psychologist, clinical social worker, family therapist, licensed counselor, or some other name sanctioned by the state, that does not give the professional the right to make a patient out of the person who walks into his office. It would be as if you walked into your accountant's office, told him of your financial troubles, and he replied, "You have the illness of bad debt! And since it is an illness, I can happily accept your medical insurance!"

The label of "patient" should be used appropriately because by its very nature it increases the power of the provider and weakens the person who is suffering. If what is present is emotional distress caused by life's problems, it is not right to apply the label of "patient." Should the very act of looking for help and walking into a certain sort of office lead to you being labeled a "patient," after which you will almost certainly be "diagnosed with a mental disorder"? It should not.

If Not "Patient," Will "Client" Do?

Sufferers who come in looking for mental health services shouldn't be labeled as patients. First, the transaction isn't a genuinely medical one, even if so-called "drugs" are often prescribed. Second, nonmedical personnel like psychologists, counselors, clinical social workers, and family therapists shouldn't have "patients." Third, the word stigmatizes the individual for no legitimate reason. There are many other good reasons, too, not to bandy about the word "patient."

But what about that most common alternative word to "patient": the word "client"? Is that a useful, appropriate word, or is that a word with its own baggage, limitations, and dangers? If we are looking to rethink mental health service provision, it is very important that we get the players in the game appropriately named. The providers should be appropriately named—we are calling them a human experience specialist. But what do we think about the word "client" for the sufferer?

Who has clients? Lawyers, accountants, high-end boutiques, real estate agents, and personal shoppers have clients. Why do plumbers have customers and personal shoppers have clients? Why do auto mechanics have customers and architects have clients? It looks like there is something about economic class built into the word "client." A bargain basement department store has customers and an expensive boutique has clients. An auto repair shop that caters to everyday cars has customers and a shop that caters to fancy cars has clients. The guests of a motel are customers and the guests of a boutique hotel are clients. If "patient" carries a tangle of meanings having to do with illness, "client" looks to come with a tangle of meanings having to do with economic class.

"Client" also appears connected to the idea of "better service." We expect that you will get "better service" or "more service" or "more personalized service" in a boutique hotel than at a motel off the highway and at a boutique dress shop rather than in the dress department of a bargain basement department store. A "cook" and a "chef" might do the same work, but from which one do we expect "better food"? By making you my client, I have made myself look better. I have instantly and effortlessly upgraded myself. Isn't that interesting? It doesn't matter whether I've done anything to merit that upgrading. Language does the trick for me!

Before we try to decide whether it makes sense to ditch such a class-driven word, one that raises the provider's status simply by how language operates, let's take a look at some alternative language. What other words exist to describe customers and consumers? Who is the customer of a parish priest? A parishioner. Who is the customer of a Zen master? A student. A cruise ship has passengers, a cab driver fares, social workers cases. None of these words or the many others words we might offer up make for a very interesting or useful alternative to "client." Are we stuck with "client" by default? Or do we perhaps have to coin some new language?

Before we think about coining any new language, however, let's look at the following issue: "customer resistance." Remember that while life is difficult, you are also difficult. We might have it in our heart to frame the relationship of the future as a certain sort of easy collaboration between sufferer and helper and maybe find a word that communicates "collaboration," but that would imply that sufferers would indeed collaborate. Would they? Let's think about that for a minute.

The Unwilling and The Unhelpful

We have to factor customer resistance into this discussion. If someone comes in wanting a pill, wanting to blame a spouse, wanting to talk but not listen, wanting insights but not the subsequent work, wanting to get better but not to change, and so on, what sort of collaboration can come from that?

We need to talk frankly. How often are human beings really interested in reducing their emotional distress? Do they always or even often really want to feel better? What if feeling better requires that you change your daily habits, change your habits of mind, change your circumstances, upgrade your personality, and work like the dickens on every aspect of your life? How many people are up for that?

A person may be suffering and may seek out a helping professional hired to help relieve emotional distress. Unfortunately for both, the sufferer may have powerful reasons for not cooperating. Maybe he doesn't want his drinking, smoking, or eating habits tampered with. Maybe he doesn't want to change—he wants the people around him to change. Maybe he's unwilling to reveal what's going on because he's embarrassed by his thoughts or his actions. Maybe there would be repercussions—say, if his mate found out about his affairs. Maybe he's very comfortable with his formed personality and his habits of mind, even though they produce sadness and anxiety.

This would make him entirely human and not very unusual. In fact, virtually all human beings prefer being who they are to being helped or to reducing their emotional distress—if being helped and reducing their distress makes work for them, requires that they change, or forces them to look in the mirror. It is an artifact of evolution that our "selfish genes" cause us to defend ourselves even against useful, life-improving help. It might prove in your best interests to make certain admissions and take a certain amount of responsibility, but most human natures rebel against this approach to life. This reality doesn't auger well for any helping relationship, present or future.

These are, of course, the sufferer's issues—but they also become the issues of the helping professional. You are forcing the person you hire to deal with human nature, and who doesn't get tired and "burn out" on human nature? The current thrust of mental health services in the direction of "diagnosing and treating mental disorders" and "medicating patients" is rooted in large measure in this tiresome transaction, that as a helper I must try to help someone who isn't helping me or himself. What psychiatrist isn't happier acting like you "have something" and writing you a prescription rather than trying to arm-wrestle you out of your personality, your habits of mind, and your ways of being? Wouldn't you be rather likely to do the same in his position?

It may be that you are more unwilling to cooperate because you have secrets to keep, or it may be that you are more unable to cooperate because your chronic sadness has drained you of the energy you need to collaborate. These are different situations, but from a helper's point of view, they amount to the same problem: you aren't helping. And that has consequences for you because your lack of cooperation will get factored into the diagnostic label you get and, in turn, will factor into your prognosis and your treatment plan.

Say that you are uncooperative—you may even be loud about it— perhaps because you have some intuitive sense that you are not going to get the help you need. The more difficult you are, the less likely you are to get some "mild" adjustment disorder diagnosis or some mood disorder diagnosis and the more likely you are to get a "severe" personality disorder diagnosis. Just as a judge has a remedy for "difficult and unpleasant" where he works—contempt of court—a therapist-as-judge has his remedy: the ability to diagnose you with a "borderline personality disorder" or an "oppositional defiant personality disorder" or something else that translates as, "Boy, you are difficult!"

This is, of course, a covert and maybe even half-unconscious operation. A psychiatrist would never say to you, "Because you are being uncooperative, I am giving you a harsher label." Nevertheless, he is likely to provide you with that harsher diagnosis for two different reasons: because he is annoyed with you and also because once he gives you that pejorative label, he is relatively off the hook as far as treating you goes. Since it is "well known" that folks with personality disorders are by-and-large unreachable and untreatable, his job has just become that much easier. A person's unwillingness to participate in reducing his own emotional distress coupled with a therapist's wish to take it easy on himself when dealing with uncooperative clients leads us to this exact moment in the history of mental health, where chemicals are running rampant and everyone acts as if human beings have caught various versions of mental flu.

It also follows that the more difficult you are, the more society will react coercively. Produce headaches for your parents and psychiatrists are waiting. The more antisocial you act, the more society will want you handled. Your screaming on the street will not be tolerated. Your suicide gesture will be criminalized. Society wants peace and quiet. Why should society's desire to protect itself surprise anyone? If you throw your pumpkin soup in the face of your waitress because you believe that she is trying to poison you, society cares about only one thing: you must stop that.

Where we have arrived is the completely predictable result of two agendas marrying: the marriage of the sufferer's wish to remain the same and the helper's wish to make it through the day. We must somehow factor this reality into any new system we devise and into our decision about how to name you. How good can any new system be if it doesn't take into account that human beings are only sometimes actually interested in reducing their emotional distress? In medicine, the issue is compliance: will a patient take his meds? Our issue is an even more intractable version of the same problem: will sufferers actually "transcend their human nature" and help themselves?

In light of these various realities, there is probably really only one thing to call you: a person. An individual who crosses a service provider's threshold is neither a patient nor a client but a person. There. We have named him. Every single other appellation confuses and obscures matters. Since only "person" captures the flavor of human obstinacy, of human resiliency—of everything human—"person" is what we must call the customer of a mental health service provider. Our human experience specialists will say, for example, "I am currently working with several people." How simple, straightforward, and truthful!

And where will that leave them? They will face the reality of difficult human beings with their tricks, adamancy, evasions, and finger pointing—that is, facing real members of our species. They aren't naïve: They expect adamancy. We respect that people who have spent a lifetime dealing with the undeniable difficulties of living will have built up protective armor. If life were easier, maybe people would defend themselves less fiercely. But it is human nature to resist change, exposure, discomfort, and so on. We are all resistant. So, while we would love it if we could propose a collaboration model as the model of the future, we must think twice about that. In such a collaboration model, the fundamental stance of helpers would change from "I am an expert with superior understanding who can diagnose you and treat you" to "I am a person with some understanding of human nature and some helping strategies who will work with you to help you frame your 'mental health' goals and achieve those goals." That is a destination we would love to arrive at; we will have to see (in future chapters) if there is a way to get there.

It matters what we call the people who visit our new human experience specialist. The name they bear is important because it helps define the nature and dynamics of the relationship. The very act of naming produces consequences. "Patient" will not do and "client" carries its own baggage. Only "person" will do. We had to get to this obvious conclusion in this laborious way because calling you a person is not customary or popular inside the mental health establishment. You yourself may have forgotten that that is who you are. When we take you to be the person you are, we can help you better. We can say, "You've been through a lot." We can ask, "Do you intend to help yourself?" We can empathize with you in all of your humanness because that is what you are, a human being. We must do this even though we find ourselves in a climate where it feels like heresy to announce that each of us is human.

6

The Mental Disorder
Labeling Fraud

It is hard to communicate the depth and breadth of the fraud currently being perpetrated on the general public by the mental heath establishment. It just doesn't seem possible that the whole mental health industry could collude in adopting a way of looking at mental health that makes no sense whatsoever. It sounds like some nutty conspiracy theory to suggest that so many smart, educated people—psychiatrists, psychologists, psychotherapists, academics, judges, etc.—would agree to perpetrate what amounts to complete fraud. It just doesn't sound possible. However, that is exactly what is going on.

The fraud is simple to describe: When we see certain things going together (and we will pick and choose which things we see and which things we refuse to see), independent of any understanding of why these things go together or whether they really go together, we will give these things a name and call them a syndrome and a mental disorder. We have no idea whatsoever what is actually going on, but by virtue of the "fact" that "these things clearly go together," we feel entitled to call them a syndrome and a mental disorder. We will base our whole mental health apparatus on this particular naming game.

This is laugh-out-loud nonsensical. It is like saying that since we see an increase in the eating of ice cream at the same time that we see an increase in paralysis, we will call what we see "ice cream paralysis disorder." That an actual disease, polio, strikes during the summer when kids eat more ice cream does not imply a connection between these two otherwise completely unconnected phenomena. The phenomena are fundamentally unconnected. Just because you "see them at the same time" is not enough to act as if they are fundamentally connected when they are only tangentially connected or not connected at all. In our crazy system, we focus as much on the "prevention of eating ice cream" as on the paralysis, and we focus not at all on the causes of the paralysis. We do not focus on causes because we currently have no understanding of the fundamental causes of or connections between the "mental health" things we observe.

In the current system, "eating ice cream" becomes a "symptom of the disorder of paralysis," and your job, since you have no idea what else to do and since a drug company has provided you with a chemical that can prevent a person from eating ice cream, is to "treat the symptom of the disorder," to get on a bandwagon to stop kids from eating ice cream, and to get home to your warm apartment. It is completely Orwellian that the bible used by the mental health establishment to "diagnose and treat mental disorders," the DSM-5, would call itself a diagnostic manual when it does not diagnose and is not a manual. It should rightly be called a Christmas catalogue for mental health professionals looking to make a profit.

The DSM names putative "mental disorders" and describes how you can "diagnose" those mental disorders based on what are called symptom pictures. It is silent on the causes of the "mental disorders" it names, and it is silent on how to treat the mental disorders it names. No doubt its producers can provide all sorts of reasons as to why they decided to fall silent on both causes and treatments, but the real reason they are silent is because the things they are describing do not exist. Suffering exists. Mental pain exists. But to be so callously and carelessly ignorant as to collect "symptoms" and to then combine those "symptoms" into "syndromes" just because an array of putative symptoms occur together (think eating ice cream and polio) is unconscionable.

Don't take my word for this. Here is Thomas Insel, director of the National Institute of Mental Health, on the subject. As part of his public announcement that the NIMH was withdrawing its support for the DSM, Insel explained, "The weakness of the manual is its lack of validity. Unlike our definitions of heart disease, lymphoma, or AIDS, the *DSM* diagnoses are based on a consensus about clusters of clinical symptoms, not any objective laboratory measure. While the *DSM* has been described as a 'Bible' for the field, it is at best a dictionary, creating a set of labels and defining each." He is likewise quoted in Gary Greenberg's *The Book of Woe*: "There is no reality to 'depression' or 'schizophrenia.' We might have to stop using terms like depression and schizophrenia because they're getting in the way."

In *Mad Science: Psychiatric Coercion, Diagnosis, and Drugs*, Stuart Kirk, Tomi Gomory, and David Cohen explain, "We will demonstrate that the touted achievements of psychiatry in the past half century including developing a novel and easily applied diagnostic approach embodied in the modern *Diagnostic and Statistical Manual of Mental Disorders (DSM)* are little more than a recycled mishmash of coercion of the mad and the misbehaving, mystification of the process of labeling people, and medical-sounding justifications for people's desire to use, and professionals' desires to give, psychoactive chemicals." Much has already been said and written over the years about the complete illegitimacy of turning "symptom pictures" into "mental disorders." But almost no one is listening, not even when the director of the National Institute of Mental Health says it.

Most people, if they have an opinion at all, believe that the "mental disorders" described in the DSM must actually exist. How could there not be things like "depression" or "schizophrenia"? How could they not exist when tens of millions of people are "diagnosed with a mental disorder" every year—including millions upon millions of children? Those "things" just must exist, mustn't they? They don't. Human suffering exists. The consequences of human suffering, like being too anxious to perform, too sad to get up and go to work, and too agitated to sleep through the night, exist. Behaviors that a parent might not like, like his child not sitting still in school, exist. Behaviors whose causes we do not understand exist by the bushel load. But their existence is not the same as the existence of "mental disorders diagnosed on the basis of symptom pictures." Why not believe the director of the National Institute of Mental Health on that score? Or at least take his opinion seriously?

It is very hard for someone not schooled in this debate to get their head around this idea that the current practice of the mental health establishment to "diagnose and treat mental disorders based on symptom pictures" is a completely illegitimate activity. To diagnose means to understand, not to observe. To see an explosion to the left and an explosion to the right does not mean that you know what has caused those explosions or whether they are connected. If you call every explosion you see "a terrorist attack," then you have created terrorist attacks simply by how you use language. When you observe something, are completely indifferent as to what is causing it, and name it something for a reason on your agenda (say, that you want more leverage to "fight terrorist attacks"), you have done something completely illegitimate. That is how the DSM operates.

It should be clear that I do not want the DSM "improved." It ought to be abandoned, and we should start over by, to begin with, telling the truth. We should say, "I don't know what caused that explosion."

We should say, "I have no idea if that explosion on the left is connected to that explosion on the right." We should say, "Let's really investigate." Many mental health professionals are currently debating whether the criteria for this or that "mental disorder" ought to be tweaked, whether this or that "mental disorder" is reliable or valid, and so on. These debates are fundamentally beside the point. The fundamental problem is that the whole enterprise is fraudulent.

The Merck Manual used by physicians to diagnose two thousand diseases and disorders addresses what causes those diseases and disorders, how to treat them, and how to prevent them. The DSM does none of that. Not a word about causes, treatment, or prevention. What does that suggest about its legitimacy? What are the implications of the fact that the DSM is silent on the causes of the disorders it names? What are the implications of the fact that the DSM is silent on how to treat the disorders it names? What are the implications of the fact that it calls itself a diagnostic manual but says "inside" that it is not really diagnosing but rather naming syndromes based on symptom pictures? The implications are that we must abandon this charade.

For more than fifty years, the Hungarian psychiatrist Thomas Szasz argued tirelessly that "mental illness" was a harmful myth and a self-serving metaphor employed by the psychiatric industry to drum up business. He wrote in *The Myth of Mental Illness*, "My aim is to suggest that the phenomena now called mental illnesses be looked at afresh and more simply, that they be removed from the category of illnesses, and that they be regarded as the expressions of man's struggle with the problem of how he should live. Since medical interventions are designed to remedy only medical problems, it is logically absurd to expect that they will help solve problems whose very existence has been defined and established on nonmedical grounds."

There is nothing new about what we who are arguing against the DSM and the medical model of mental illness are saying. It has been said before, smartly and eloquently, and has fallen on deaf ears decade after decade. But maybe this is a new day and a new moment. So in that spirit, let's continue our discussion by looking at three related follies: imagining that mental disorders exist just because the phrase "mental disorder" can be defined; calling indicators of human experience "symptoms of mental disorders" and collecting those "symptoms" into "symptom pictures" called "syndromes"; and designating the book in which those pictures appear a manual and not, as it ought properly to be called, a mere catalogue.

Defining a Mental Disorder Does Not Make it Exist

Defining a made-up thing or naming the attributes of a made-up thing does not make that thing exist. Naming the attributes of a made-up god—that he is all loving, all knowing, vengeful, in charge of the tides, five-headed, etc.—does not make a made-up god exist. Naming the attributes of a unicorn—that it must have one horn and not two or that it must stand on four legs and not five—does not make it exist. Defining god as all loving or a unicorn as a one-horned creature does not make either exist. Defining a mental disorder does not make a mental disorder exist. There is nothing easier than defining things: defining is child's play. That something appears in a dictionary because it can be defined does not make that thing real.

No one doubts the phenomena of birds and bees. But to call birds and bees miracles and to create a miracle-maker god who created them is a certain kind of fraudulent leap. One shouldn't move from birds and bees to gods just because language allows you to do so. Similarly, no one really doubts the phenomena of sadness, worry, agitation, rage, confusion, and so on. But to call these phenomena symptoms of mental disorders is exactly the same sort of fraudulent leap. We make gods and mental disorders in exactly the same fraudulent way: by illegitimately using real phenomena as "proof" of the existence of nonexisting things.

Part of the joy and ease of this fraudulent creating is that you can define the nonexisting thing any way you like. Who is to say if a god is or isn't friendly, spiteful, eternal, or taking a personal interest in you if there is no real thing involved? If there is no real thing involved, who is to say if a mental disorder is the same or different from a brain disorder; the same or different for a Jungian, a Freudian, or a chemical dispenser; the same or different from unwanted thoughts or behaviors? It ought to be the case that those making the claim for a nonexisting thing should have to prove its existence, but in real life the burden always falls on the whistle-blower. The perpetrators have it easy!

See how blissfully easy the definers of nonexisting mental disorders have it. First they define "mental disorder" one way, as they did in the DSM-4: "A mental disorder is a clinically significant behavioral or psychological syndrome or pattern that occurs in an individual and that is associated with present distress or disability or with a significantly increased risk of suffering death, pain, disability, or an important loss of freedom." If you pay attention and spend the time, you will discern that this says nothing in particular. But our interest for the moment is in the following funny event: the ease with which they ditched this definition and replaced it with another one in the DSM-5.

Under pressure by skeptics as to the whether this definition made any sense whatsoever, the American Psychiatric Association redefined nonexisting mental disorders a new way in the DSM-5: "A mental disorder is a syndrome characterized by clinically significant disturbance in an individual's cognition, emotion regulation, or behavior that reflects a dysfunction in the psychological, biological, or developmental processes underlying mental functioning. Mental disorders are usually associated with significant distress in social, occupational, or other important activities. An expectable or culturally approved response to a common stressor or loss, such as the death of a loved one, is not a mental disorder. Socially deviant behavior (e.g., political, religious, or sexual) and conflicts that are primarily between the individual and society are not mental disorders unless the deviance or conflict results from a dysfunction in the individual, as described above."

Forget for a moment what this definition seems to be saying. The very idea that you can radically change the definition of something without anything in the real world changing and with no new increases in knowledge or understanding is at first glance remarkable—remarkable until you realize that the thing being defined does not exist. It is completely easy—effortless, really—to change the definition of something that does not exist to suit your current purposes. In fact, there is hardly any better proof of the nonexistence of a nonexisting thing than that you can define it one way today, another way tomorrow, and a third way on Sunday.

If you had the patience and the interest, you might want to scrutinize the changes made to the definition of a "mental disorder" and come to your own personal understanding of how language has been employed here to cover all bases, support societal goals, and say absolutely nothing about human reality. A mental disorder is a psychological thing—or maybe it isn't. A mental disorder is a biological thing—or maybe it isn't. You can rail against your society unless you have a "dysfunction," at which point your railing is a mental disorder. You can disagree with your politicians unless you have a "dysfunction," at which point you are a mental deviant. One could go on and on making such observations, and yet making such observations actually plays into the hands of the creators of nonexisting things, who love it if you play their game. They can slip about with impunity, adding, qualifying, and shifting, while you waste your breath being reasonable and thoughtful.

The question is not, "What is the best definition of a mental disorder?" The question is not, "Is the DSM-5 definition of a mental disorder better than the DSM-4 definition of a mental disorder?" Those are absolutely not the right questions! The first and only question is, "Do mental disorders exist?" The phenomena of sadness, worry, pain, distress, angst, and so on exist. Just as the birds and bees exist, pain and suffering exist. But birds do not prove the existence of gods and pain does not prove the existence of mental disorders. Let us not play the game of debating the definitions of nonexistent things. Let us move right on!

Let's take one further brief moment to look at another slippery place: the definitions of "mental health." We will come back to this in a future chapter since the matter is really of great importance. Just as it matters a great deal what the phrase "mental disorder" actually stands for, it matters a great deal what the phrase "mental health" stands for. For now, and while we're on the subject of defining nonexisting things into "definitional existence," let's look at how the idea of "mental health" is defined into existence. Here are some commonly employed dictionary definitions of "mental health":

"Mental health is a state of emotional and psychological well-being in which an individual is able to use his or her cognitive and emotional capabilities, function in society, and meet the ordinary demands of everyday life." In this view you are abnormal or unhealthy (as opposed, for example, to despairing or stressed out) if you are unable to meet the ordinary demands of everyday life.

"Mental health is a person's overall emotional and psychological condition." What does that mean? Could a sentence say less?

"Mental health describes a level of psychological well-being or an absence of a mental disorder." Mental health is the absence of a mental disorder?

Here is the definition of mental health as employed by the World Health Organization: "Mental health is defined as a state of well-being in which every individual realizes his or her own potential, can cope with the normal stresses of life, can work productively and fruitfully, and is able to make a contribution to her or his community." Have you ever heard a less psychological and more social definition of mental health than that? Can't you just feel the coercion coming if and when you refuse to "make a contribution to your community"?

Phrases like "mental health" and "mental disorder" matter a lot. They must not be idly defined into existence. It is one thing if there is no such thing as a "mental disorder"—that is a huge deal. But just as huge a deal is the possibility that there are multiple varieties of "mental health"—or rather, nothing that really resembles "mental health" but rather different ways of looking at human reality such that an aware person might say to himself, "You know, *this* is what I think I mean by mental health and *this* is what I would like to achieve for myself." Such concepts as "mental disorder" and "mental health" have to make more than definitional sense—they have to make real sense. Right now they do not.

The Folly of "Mental Disorder" Symptom Pictures

When you illegitimately define something like a "mental disorder" into existence, you then need to operationalize that definition so that you have a way of further "recognizing" this nonexisting thing. If you invent a unicorn, you then have to announce how many horns it has and how many feet it has. In our current system, having turned genuine human distress into "mental disorders" by definition, the next step is to "describe" these "mental disorders." This is done via what is known as "symptom pictures," a lovely phrase pulled from the world of medicine to make this illegitimate naming game sound more scientific, medical, and believable.

Our current mental health system is organized around the idea of symptoms and the idea of collections of symptoms called symptom pictures. This is its fundamental orientation. All the mental disorders that the DSM catalogues are described in terms of symptom pictures and not in terms of possible causes or sources of the "disorder" or in terms of any underlying logic. You are never told why this collection of "symptoms" should be called this "disorder." The unstated premise is that each "symptom picture" is an accurate description of a real thing and somehow amounts to that real thing. No reasons are given for this assumption, though something about the title of DSM—the "statistical" part—is supposed to suggest that this is somehow a "statistical matter."

If a mental disorder were something like an actual illness, disease, or disorder, both you and the person who treats you would want more than a symptom picture—you would want to know what was going on. You would want an explanation. A symptom picture is not an explanation. That symptom pictures alone are used to "diagnose mental disorders" should cause you to jump out of your chair and exclaim, "Wow, that *is* alarming!" To repeat: a symptom picture is not an explanation. Your hands might be rough because you have a skin problem or because you lay bricks. Dabbing on an ointment may make the symptom of roughness go away whether it is caused by an ailment or by your job, but if the roughness is caused by an ailment that really requires further treatment, then the opportunity to know what that ailment is has been missed.

The same is true in the diagnosing and treating of so-called mental disorders. The chemicals you receive may alleviate some, many, or all of your symptoms, such that you are able to report that you "feel better." But if it is profound unhappiness that has caused the "symptoms" and not a biological disorder, what do you suppose are the chances that you are really "cured"? Zero. You have been "put in another state," not treated. We will look at this difference in detail in the next chapter, but the main idea is that just because you get a psychiatric label based on a symptom picture and are prescribed chemicals that then have a "positive effect" on you does not mean that you have been genuinely "diagnosed and treated." It only looks that way!

Let's say that you find yourself sitting inert for hours at a time in front of your television set eating potato chips, not speaking to the people around you, refusing to clean your apartment, and barely dragging yourself to work. A psychiatrist looks at that "symptom picture" and says that you're obviously depressed and that you ought to go on an antidepressant right now. What if what is actually going on is that you received some scathing criticism at work that sent your world reeling and your sense of yourself plummeting and that you haven't begun to recover from that blow yet? The symptom picture without an explanation only gets you chemicals. The appropriate explanation makes sense of your unhappiness and alerts you as to what you might need to do to recover: change your job, build your self-confidence, and so on.

When you rely on symptom pictures rather than explanations to "diagnose" human challenges and when you create "treatments" intended to reduce or eliminate the "symptoms" rather than addressing the human issues involved, it is not far-fetched to imagine a time when the clerk at your local big box store will be empowered to scan a laundry list of "symptoms," check them off, and send you to a counter at the back of the store where a busy pharmacist will dispense the antidepressant of the month. This is a simple affair, using a checklist to pin on a label, and we are heading in the direction of everyone everywhere taking psychiatric chemicals to "treat" one or another of a huge laundry list of "mental disorders."

"Symptom" is a medical word and should be reserved for medicine. Your low energy might be a symptom of a thyroid condition or an indicator that you aren't getting enough sleep. If it happened to be the latter, you would go to bed earlier and see what happened. If it happened to be the former, you would seek medical attention. This is a difference that matters! It matters whether something we observe is a symptom of a medical condition or an indicator of a life situation. Your current sadness could be an indicator that you hate your job, that your mate is critical of you, that you are having trouble paying your bills, that you are realizing none of your dreams, that you were born sad, and so on. But of what medical condition could it be a symptom? What medical condition produces sadness?

This is a different question from what medical condition might make you feel sad because you have it. Almost any might do that! We have to get clear on this distinction if we have any chance at better mental health. There is a difference between a medical condition "producing sadness" as a biological byproduct of its processes and us "feeling sad" as a psychological matter because we have a medical condition. In the latter case, our sadness is an indicator of a human experience and not a symptom of a medical disorder. What medical condition causes anger, irritability, boredom, euphoria, awe, love, or anything else, positive or negative, that human beings feel? If you say to me, well, a brain tumor might cause fits of irrational anger and epileptic fits are often preceded by a feeling like euphoria, I would reply, yes! Now we are making the correct connection between an organic problem and what we're observing. Yes! This is what diagnosing means.

We will return to this matter of cause and effect in human affairs in a later chapter. For now, let me repeat our headline. When you define mental disorders into existence, you then need to create a way to recognize them. This fraudulent "recognizing" is done nowadays through the device and ruse of so-called symptom pictures.

Manual or Catalogue?

To repeat: *The Diagnostic and Statistical Manual of Mental Disorders* provides no diagnoses and isn't a manual. A manual tells you how to do something. The DSM tells you how to do nothing except put a label on a picture. That is what catalogues do: they provide you with a picture of a sofa, give the sofa a name (like "craftsman sectional"), and add some details so that you can make a purchase. In this regard, the DSM is precisely a catalogue that allows mental health practitioners to make sales and not a manual that tells them how to do something. A genuine manual of mental disorders would tell you how to treat those mental disorders. A pretty catalogue of pictures and labels need do no such thing.

A manual has utility. The logic of a manual is that you get instructions for doing something. These instructions go beyond just naming things. An engine manual not only names the parts of an engine but tells you what to do when a certain red light comes on or when you hear a certain grinding noise as you drive. A manual of any sort does more than just name, it instructs and explains. A catalogue, on the other hand, just names and describes things. It may put the named and described things into categories, like glassware, silverware, and small appliances, it may even make some connections among items, for example, presenting how a living room ensemble might come together from items in the sofa section, the table section, and the lamp section. But its goal is to sell you things, not to instruct you.

A manual is for understanding and a catalogue is for shopping. The DSM is a holiday catalogue for mental health professionals and not a manual of instruction. A genuine mental health manual would present various hypotheses about the sources of emotional distress. Given our limited understanding, it might have to call these guesses or best guesses rather than hypotheses. If it were felt that not enough was known about our species to hypothesize or even make guesses about the sources and causes of emotional distress, it would say so. This hypothesizing might sound like, "Anxiety is a normal feature of our species. It is an aspect of our warning system against danger. It appears that some people suffer from more anxiety than other people do. Here are some thoughts on why that might be the case."

These thoughts and speculations might sound like, "In a hereditary model, excessive anxiety is conceptualized as a. In a biological model, excessive anxiety is conceptualized as b. In a cognitive-behavioral model, excessive anxiety is conceptualized as c. From a self-psychological standpoint, excessive anxiety is conceptualized as d. A Jungian might conceptualize excessive anxiety as e." And so on. It would present many theoretical perspectives on excessive anxiety while clearly articulating that none of them have been adequately researched. Most or all of these "theoretical perspectives" might amount to nothing more than opinions and guesses. Nevertheless, such a manual would at least paint a true picture of our current understanding, as limited as it might be, of phenomena like excessive anxiety.

Attempts of this sort would amount to beginning efforts toward a genuine manual of emotional health rather than our current mere catalogue of putative mental disorders. In our future genuine manual, if we knew enough to be able to do so, we would want to add the following two refinements. First, we would want to rank order these so-to-speak reasons, saying something like, "Limited research seems to indicate that most excessive anxiety is probably of the hereditary sort. Other quite limited research suggests that the second most usual source of excessive anxiety is cognitive distortions. The third most usual source of excessive anxiety seems to be such-and-such," and so on. We are certainly nowhere near being able to say such things at the present time; if we could, that would be really helpful.

A second refinement would be to express how excessive anxiety might manifest itself depending on its source. This might sound like, "If the source of the excessive anxiety is existential in nature, you would expect it to manifest most prominently in circumstances that seem to the individual very important, like a seminal audition or performance for a musician, since at such times life purpose and life meaning are involved. However, if cognitive distortions were causing the excessive anxiety, then we would expect the anxiety to generalize and flare up in small matters as well as large matters—maybe even more powerfully in small matters." And so on. We do not know such things now, and it may be impossible to ever know such things; if we did know them, that would prove extremely useful.

A genuine manual would then continue with treatment options and present the rationale for its suggestions. It would indicate when and why you would want to use chemicals, when and why you would want to use one form of talk therapy versus another form of talk therapy, and when and why you would want to make other sorts of suggestions and try other sorts of things. If it were possible to do so, you would want to continue in the following vein: "With a cognitive approach, you might expect the following positive effects, the following negative effects, and also no effects in certain instances. You should expect a cognitive approach to have limited or no effect on excessive anxiety if the source of that anxiety is genetic but significant effect if it is learned," and so on.

This is one way a genuine mental health manual might sound. The DSM is certainly not this sort of manual. Part of the vital enterprise of rethinking mental health involves thinking through how we might move from mere catalogue to actual manual. This task may prove impossible, but perhaps there is enough known that a beginning attempt could be made. A catalogue of putative mental disorders is not the same thing as an actual treatment manual. Providers need either a genuine treatment manual, a beginning version of such a treatment manual, or else clear guidelines about what to do in the absence of such a treatment manual. We will return to this theme in future chapters.

7

Chemicals versus Medication

In the future, if we are wise enough to look this distinction in the eye, we will begin to understand the difference between chemicals with effects and medications that treat illnesses. Currently we are not that wise. We carelessly call a chemical a drug even if it is not treating a disorder or a disease. By so doing, we play right into the hands of the mental health establishment, the folks who want us to think that the chemicals-with-effects that they wantonly prescribe are legitimate medicine. They are surely chemicals-with-effects, effects that you may indeed want, but they are not medication employed for the treatment of actual disorders. Not when the "disorder" is the hatred of your job, your collapsing relationship, your high intelligence, or your existential dismay!

Medicine is wonderful. But the chemicals employed to "treat mental disorders" are not medicine. Not every chemical used by a person to create an effect can rightly be called medicine. If we use language this loosely and call every chemical with a powerful effect a medicine, then we have completely bastardized language and made a mockery of the ideas of disease and of medication. Biologically altering our experience of life via chemicals is not the same as treating illnesses with drugs. If we are not adamant in our defense of this distinction, then every single chemical compound is raised by loose language to the special status of medication.

Human beings have used chemicals to alter their experience of life since the beginning of time: peyote, magic mushrooms, Scotch, marijuana, cocaine, nicotine, caffeine, heroin, red wine. The list of chemicals used by human beings for the purpose of feeling different is very long. It is only metaphoric—and a profoundly dangerous and ill-chosen metaphor—to call these "medications that treat the disease of life." You can call these chemicals sacred, dangerous, a blessing, a problem, or whatever else you like, but don't call them medicine.

A chemical becomes medicine in context. *It changes its name by virtue of how it is being used.* The chemicals called antibiotics are being used to treat your infection. They are still "mere" chemicals but they have been legitimately elevated to the high status of medication by virtue of why and how they are being used. We call them medicine because they are being used to treat an actual disease. If the disease were not there—if we were not using these chemicals to fight something worse than the chemicals themselves—we would not subject anyone to those powerful chemicals.

Three problems conspire to make our conversations about mental health and medication problematic. First is the completely loose way that we use the word "drug." It would help us tremendously if we reserved the word "drug" or "medication" or "medicine" for those times when we used a certain chemical to treat a particular ailment, malady, injury, disorder, or disease. In order to use the word "drug" or "medication" there would need to be a direct relationship between the chemical and the disorder. Only then would the chemical rise to the status of "medicine." Two things would be required: that there is a disorder and that the chemical directly affects it.

If there is no disorder to treat, you can't call the chemical you take "medicine." Just as it would be useful to reserve the word "drug" or "medication" or "medicine" for those times that a chemical was used to treat an actual disorder, it would be useful not to make up disorders that do not exist. Cancer is one thing, and "communism as a cancer of the mind" is another thing. The first is a medical condition; the second is a metaphor. If you drink vodka to get over your enthusiasm for communism, in that transaction vodka is not "medication" and your enthusiasm for communism is not "a mental disorder." Vodka is not medication and can't be medication in this instance, not because it is a mere chemical, but because there is no disorder present except metaphorically.

Marijuana is a substance. It is a mere chemical-with-effects when we use it to alter our experience of reality, and it is medicine if we use it as treatment for our glaucoma. Glaucoma is a certain identifiable medical condition and not a metaphor. "Life sucks" is a certain existential or psychological issue, real in its pain but not a medical condition. Smoking marijuana to "leave life for a bit" is not a "treatment" of anything medical but rather a characteristic use of a certain chemical substance to alter our experience of reality. If we could reserve "drug," "medication," or "medicine" as words that we only use when we are talking about treating actual biological disorders, it would amount to a giant step forward.

It would be lovely if we could also get the following distinctions made. There ought to be a way to language the difference between treating a disorder, treating a symptom of a disorder, using a chemical for some purpose while trying to treat a disorder, and treating something we mistakenly call "a symptom of a disorder" when no disorder exists. These are four distinct situations that are currently crushed together as one. To understand what I mean, consider the following scenario.

Sally is affected by a serious bacterial infection that is hard to eradicate. She takes antibiotics to treat the bacterial infection. In our naming scheme, we are happy to call the antibiotics she is taking "drugs used to treat a biological ailment."

Say that her infection produces a rash that can be reduced by the application of a topical ointment. What shall we call the rash? On the one hand, it is a "symptom" of the bacterial infection and might even have been used to diagnose the presence of the bacterial infection. On the other hand, it is a certain sort of "result" of the infection. In this context, it is quite fair to call that topical ointment a drug, and its use a treatment for either a symptom or a result of the infection.

Now say that her infection also makes sleep difficult. Her insomnia is not precisely a symptom of her bacterial infection, but it is the result of her bacterial infection—if, of course, that is what ails her. It could also be the result of something else. Say that Sally is given a sedative or some other chemical to deal with the insomnia. In this case, the chemical is not a drug to treat the infection and it is not a drug to treat a symptom of the infection. It is something else again—and we could give it a name like "ancillary medication" or something along those lines.

Remember that in this scenario we believe there is a direct connection between the insomnia and the infection. We believe the infection, rather than worries about the infection or worries about something else, is causing the insomnia. In this scenario there is still direct linkage between the infection and the insomnia. But we are beginning to skate on thin ice here; it is hard to see how we could know for sure what is causing the insomnia. Nevertheless, let's grant the chemicals in this instance the exalted title of medicine—even though we are a little leery of doing so.

Say that the chronic nature of the infection starts to make Sally sad. Now we have to be really careful about what we call the chemicals she is given. She has no sudden "mental disorder"—rather, she is bitterly sad that she can't shake this infection. If she sees a mental health practitioner, her sadness will be transformed into the "mental disorder of depression." As a result of the "diagnosis" of a "clinical depression," she will get a chemical-with-an-effect known as an "antidepressant" to "treat" what is a fictitious disorder. This is the place where we really do not want to call a chemical medicine.

Sally would probably say that she was on four medications, antibiotics for her infection, a topical for her rash, a sedative for her insomnia, and an antidepressant for her depression. She is not trained or helped to make the distinctions I've just been making. Because she isn't likely to be able to make these distinctions, she isn't able to see that the antidepressant has snuck in there as medication when, since it is not treating a disorder, not treating a symptom of a disorder, and not ancillary to the treatment of a disorder, it is really a chemical-with-an-effect. She may want that effect, but she is taking three medications and not four.

Remember Jim from our earlier discussion of diagnosing—the fellow who had suddenly become extremely anxious? His sudden anxiety may have been brought on by his scary flight home from his trip, from his conflicted feelings about the affair he has just begun, from his fear of his impending audit, or for some other reason or combination of reasons. That he has recently become anxious does not mean that he suddenly has a "mental disorder." If he doesn't suddenly have a mental disorder—if, for example, his anxiety is a product of his conflicted feelings about his extramarital affair—then any "anti-anxiety medication" he may be prescribed can't properly be called medication for a mental disorder, medication for a symptom of a mental disorder, or medication ancillary to a mental disorder. It is simply a powerful chemical being used to alter Jim's experience of life.

But isn't Jim going to think that he is now "under a doctor's treatment" for a "mental disorder" and "on medication"? In fact what has happened is that he has gone to a chemical dispenser who has no idea why Jim is anxious and who has no real curiosity about why Jim is anxious but knows that he has chemicals to dispense. Since there is no genuine diagnosing going on, no genuine mental disorder present, and no dispensing of genuine medication, it is no wonder that these interactions take only ten or fifteen minutes nowadays. They take only slightly longer than wandering into a natural food shop to find an herb or into a liquor store to grab a bottle of Scotch.

Getting this distinction straight is important. Would you buy that the word "medicine" has been appropriately used in any of the following cases? From a killer: "Arsenic is the medicine I use to treat the disease of being alive from which my victims regularly suffer." From a safari guide: "Tranquilizer darts are the medicine I use to treat the animals I encounter who are suffering from the disease of wanting to eat me." From a bar patron: "Scotch is the medicine I use to treat my disease of having a wife I can't stand." Would you accept any of those usages?

If a mental health establishment worker makes no effort to identify the cause of your suffering and is completely indifferent as to whether you are suffering from a life problem, a feature of your formed personality, a feature of your original personal, a reaction to your circumstances, a biological onslaught, a psychological issue, etc.—makes zero effort and simply says, "We call your symptom picture a mental disorder and we medicate it," you should treat his utterance with as much disdain as you treat the utterances of the poisoner, the safari guide, and the bar patron.

That isn't to say that you may not want what the psychiatrist is offering. The bar patron may get value from his Scotch. The safari guide may get great, life–saving value from his tranquilizer darts. You may want a certain effect even if you have no mental disorder. You may want a tranquilizer to deal with anxiety even if you don't have "generalized anxiety." You might also decide that you don't want that tranquilizer. You may want a mood-altering substance to deal with your chronic sadness even if you don't have "clinical depression." You might also decide that you don't want that mood-altering substance. If a chemical is available that has a certain powerful effect that you desire (and if you believe that it really has that effect and that its positive value outweighs its risks), then the chemical is yours for the taking.

Just don't think of those chemicals as "medicine." If your mental health provider is unable or unwilling to distinguish between suffering arising from a life problem, a feature of your formed personality, a reaction to your circumstances, a psychological issue, and so on, versus a biologically-based "illness" or "disorder" where the word "medicine" would be applicable, then you should feel confident that you are being prescribed chemicals and not medicine. Vodka is one thing and insulin is another. We must not let linguistic slippage confuse one with the other.

Here is how the above discussion might sound as a bit of Socratic dialogue.

"If you stub your toe, you've stubbed your toe. Yes?"
"Yes."
"And if it hurts, you can take a painkiller to ease the pain. Yes?"
"Yes."

"But the painkiller is not 'treating' your stubbed-toe-ness, yes?"

"I'm not sure."

"Let's take another example. Say that you have cancer. You're at the end of your life, and we can't effectively treat the cancer any longer. We are no longer treating the cancer, yes?"

"Yes."

"But I can say to you, 'We can give you painkillers to make your last days easier.' That's clear, yes?"

"Yes."

"Those painkillers are not treating the cancer, yes?"

"Yes!"

"So you can see the difference between diagnosing and treating your cancer and giving you a chemical for some associated reason, like reducing your pain?"

"I think I can see that."

"Okay! And so you can also see the logic of reserving the word 'drug' or 'medicine' for those times when we have diagnosed a disorder or disease and are using a certain substance to treat that disorder or disease and refusing to use the words 'drug' or 'medicine' in other instances where we haven't diagnosed a disorder or disease and aren't actively treating a disorder or disease?"

"I think I can see the logic of that reservation. But is it really necessary? Are we that confused on the issue? And does it really matter?"

"It matters a great deal! When you get an anesthetic so that surgery can be performed, it is called an anesthetic for a reason, so as to distinguish it from drugs used to treat an ailment. Technically, you are being 'anesthetized' and not 'drugged.' That may only sound of linguistic interest. But what if your antidepressant is not a 'drug for the mental disorder of depression' but 'an anesthetic to anesthetize your sadness'? If it was really the latter, you would suddenly understand that you are not being treated but anesthetized—and that's a big difference, isn't it?"

"That is a big difference!"

I have asked you throughout this book to notice how language is used and abused by the mental health establishment. We are once again back concerning ourselves with the power and importance of language because it is through the clever use of language that the mental health establishment is foisting powerful chemicals on unsuspecting sufferers—on millions of adults and on millions of children, too. Phenomena exist—sadness, anxiety, irritability, distractibility, etc. These phenomena are transformed through labeling into "mental disorders," then "treated" with so-called "medicine." This is simple to say but very hard to combat.

Walking a Line

What is our human experience specialist to do with this difficult conundrum, that "psychiatric medications" are only chemicals-with-effects but that many human beings may want the powerful effects these chemicals afford? Trying to explain this matter clearly to the people she helps might actually put the specialist at risk, given that the current standard of care is based on the idea of "diagnosing mental disorders" and, once diagnosed, "treating" them with "drugs."

There are three camps in the mental health field with respect to so-called psychiatric medications: those who prescribe and advocate for them, whether or not they fully believe in them; those who believe that so-called psychiatric medications are something rather different from medicine—namely chemicals with powerful effects—and who see some place for those powerful effects if only their rationale were differently presented; and those who prefer to stay as far away from the fray as possible, using other methods (like talk) to help their clients and remaining mute on this particular controversy.

A human experience specialist falls in the second camp. Put yourself in this role. As a human experience specialist, you believe that we don't understand the human situation, the human mind, and human affairs well enough to really know what is going on when a person complains of chronic sadness or chronic anxiety, mutters to himself, hoards, looks eccentric, or makes online purchases from dawn to dusk with no need for the items purchased. We could name fifty possible causes for what we're seeing without, however, having much of a way of narrowing those causes down or knowing which, if any, were personality-driven, psychological, circumstantial, genetic, biological, or "medical" in nature.

As a human experience specialist, you would like mental health professionals to admit, as you are bravely doing, that it is quite beyond us to know what is causing or compelling these sorts of experiences, states of being, and behaviors. You would like it further announced that we are at a seriously unfortunate place in our relation to this genuine not-knowing: instead of admitting that we do not know, we in fact claim to know and by rhetorical means turn each of these pictures, whatever is causing it, and whatever it "really" is, into a "mental disorder." We then claim to have "medicine" that effectively "treats" these "mental disorders."

You believe that we are currently fibbing when we assert that we know. You believe that what we have instead is a deep lack of knowledge. You further believe that what we currently possess are chemicals with strong effects, some of which can reasonably be considered positive and some of which must certainly be considered negative, effects able to alter our experience of life rather than treat any so-called mental disorder. You would like to share your understanding with the human beings you work with and let them know about these chemicals and their relative pluses and minuses. Do you dare, given that virtually everyone else is acting as if these are genuine medications?

You can, of course, express your opinions in print—I am doing that here. But what if you want to share your opinions with an actual human being sitting across from you? What is the right, smart, best, or safest thing to do in that situation, given that the person you are working with might benefit from the chemical in question, its downside notwithstanding? While we wait for a different future, one where our lack of knowledge is generally admitted, where opinions of this sort are safe to share, and where, perhaps, a new, extensive research project has been launched that moves our understanding forward, what can a practitioner in this position do right now?

Let's imagine how you might proceed with a fellow we'll call Bill who is complaining of, among other things, confusion, an inability to concentrate, and a lot of sadness. At a certain point—when, we'll discuss in a moment—you might want to say to Bill, "You know, a psychiatrist could provide you with chemicals that may well change your experience of life. Would you like to look into that?"

"Gee! Great!" Bill exclaims. "So you mean that you have medicine that can treat my depression and my attention deficit disorder?"

"No, unfortunately not," you must reluctantly reply. "We have no idea what's going on inside of you and really can't legitimately call what you're presenting as disorders or illnesses. It might be anything under the sun—something about your personality, something about your circumstances, something about your relationship to life purpose and meaning, something about a particular stressor, something biological, something psychological, and so on—we don't know, do we? We don't know what it is or what to call it. But we have some evidence—actually some hotly disputed evidence—that when a person presents the picture you're presenting, certain chemicals that psychiatrists have at their disposal can change that person's experience of life. Was that clear?"

"Golly, not at all."

"I can try to explain it again. Would you like me to do that?"

"No, no, no!" Bill forlornly holds his head. He has a thought. "And . . . would there be side effects to these . . . chemicals?"

"Of course."

"Well, what's the likelihood that these . . . chemicals . . . would actually help?"

"Here's a handout on that. It's a very complicated, uncertain, and disputed area. I would say that the chemical in question has some chance of changing your experience of life."

"Gee. I'm not at all sure what to do with what you're telling me. 'Change my experience of life.' I just want what I'm feeling to go away."

"I know. It's complicated."

How unsatisfying is this conversation! And how dangerous as well! How much do you want to have that conversation? How much trust and rapport would that build? The mental health establishment, which includes the courts, is entrenched in such a way that to expose it is to expose you to risk. The truth might ultimately prove a sufficient defense: many cases have been won against psychiatrists, mental institutions, drugs companies, and other members of the mental health establishment. But defending yourself is a long trip down a bad road.

We would like our human experience specialist to be permitted to say her piece, even if it is complicated and unsatisfactory. Therefore we would like her to be legally immunized to tell this truth. It should not have to prove legally dangerous to call these chemicals-with-powerful-effects what they are just because there is a standard of care mythology that calls them "medicine." But there is that standard of care mythology, and all of the power and leverage are on the side of the mental health establishment. It would not matter how many fellow thinkers in the critical psychiatry movement or patients' rights movement you could line up to support your contention. Their support would not inoculate you from risk.

It should be obvious how important it is that we say these things and speak our piece. If we stay silent, we promote the creation of more chemicals-with-powerful-effects. Do we want a powerful chemical that will excite us when we're bored (in addition, of course, to the illegal street chemicals already available for that purpose), one that will be advertised as "treating the mental disorder of chronic boredom syndrome?" Do we want a powerful chemical that will counteract our recognition of mortality, some immortality drug better than religion that provides us with an immortality fix and that can be administered as "treating the mental disorder of mortophobia?" It will prove child's play for pharmaceutical companies to come up with endless chemicals-with-powerful-effects for every possible human experience. Do we want to continue racing down that road without anyone objecting?

If, despite the risks involved, you nevertheless decide to engage in this difficult conversation, when would you have it? If you are a practitioner who has decided to stay out of the fray and who works exclusively by some other method like talking, body work or movement, you might postpone it indefinitely—maybe it won't even enter your head to bring it up. If, however, you are a human experience specialist, then it is on your shoulders to decide whether to bring the matter up sooner or later. To the extent that you don't much believe in the chemical approach you'll be inclined to postpone having this conversation in order to give your other "interventions" a chance to work. However, if Bill is in a seriously distressed state, including, for example, a suicidal one, you will probably be inclined to have the conversation early. Which "time" will you choose? Is this a "first session" conversation, an "as needed" conversation, or what?

Compounding the problem is the following. Can a person who is severely sad or intensely anxious or invested in believing that he has a mental disorder really be expected to listen to your complicated explanations or know what to do when handed this confusing choice? Can even a highly educated, relatively undisturbed person calmly contemplate such an uncomfortable choice? Imagine your surgeon saying to you, "Surgery may be a really terrible idea with only some slight likelihood of a positive outcome. So, would you like to have the surgery?" Wouldn't such a message make you highly anxious and terribly confused and put you completely out of sorts? Human beings in distress want to hear, "We have something to treat that." They want to hear that and not long stories about complicated reality.

If you are tracking the logic of my argument, you will have realized that in the future there would be no more diagnosing of mental disorders or diseases, not until a whole generation of untainted new researchers applied themselves to the question of what, if anything, the construct "mental disorder" or "mental illness" could legitimately be construed to mean. Until that time, there would be no more talk of treating "mental disorders" or "mental disease" with chemicals or with anything else. Rather, a chemical-oriented practitioner (that is, a psychiatrist) would be obliged to say, "Here's a chemical to stop the voices," "Here's a chemical to alter your mood," "Here's a chemical to tranquilize your anxiety," and so on. A psychiatrist would still have chemicals to dispense but would start telling the truth.

If this new generation of honest researchers concluded that the phrases "mental disorder" and "mental illness" could not properly be resurrected or resuscitated, then we would have a diagnosis-free future. It would naturally follow that no "medicine" could any longer be offered up as "treatment" for all those now defunct labels. Instead, psychiatrists would have "chemical repositories," maybe not unlike liquor stores, where they dispensed chemicals-with-powerful-effects whose effects changed moods, tranquilized anxiety, slowed a racing brain, silenced voices, and so on. New ads would sound like this: "Feeling sad? We have a chemical to alter your mood!" "Feeling anxious? We have a chemical to force calmness on you!"

This chapter hasn't been about whether so-called psychiatric medicine works or doesn't work, to what extent the side effects of psychiatric medicine outweigh their possible benefits, or whether you should take them or not take them. It has been about the extent to which mental disorders are created fictions that take painful or unwanted human phenomena and label them by committee as one thing or another. Exactly to that extent must so-called psychiatric medication be called chemicals-with-powerful-effects and not medicine.

If you don't believe in the legitimacy of the current labeling system, you should also not believe in a labeling system that elevates a given chemical to the high status of medicine. In the better future I have in mind, these chemicals, and more like them that are no doubt coming, might still be available and might prove helpful to some. They just wouldn't be called medicine. Their logic would become completely exposed, and new, better conversations about their use or avoidance would prove possible.

8

On Meds

Here are seven actual stories of human experiences to help flesh out the ideas expressed in the previous chapter. These stories are not meant to prove or disprove anything with respect to so-called psychiatric medications. I presented my arguments in the last chapter in that regard, and I am not intending that these stories serve as evidence one way or the other. Rather, I simply want to show the human face of living "on meds" after receiving a mental disorder diagnosis. Some of these stories have been shortened from longer narratives but they are all otherwise untouched. These are snapshots of the present state of mental health treatment.

These folks are suffering either from what is nowadays called "clinical depression" or from what is nowadays called "bipolar disorder" (formerly manic-depression). I could have added stories of folks on meds for anxiety disorders, attention deficit disorders, and so on; there are scores of "mental disorders" currently being "treated with psychoactive medication," including the many "mental disorder" labels handed children. But this chapter isn't meant to serve as a cross-section or do justice to the tens of millions of folks on psychiatric meds. Rather it is provided to put a human face on our discussion.

Barbara

I had been severely depressed even as a child since I was sexually abused by a parent and mentally abused by both my parents, whom now I totally recognize as mentally ill. I also suffered PTSD when I had married a Mormon man at seventeen to get away from the abuse, and he turned out to be an equal abuser. He literally kidnapped my three children, and I did not see them again for some twenty-eight years when I managed to find my daughter.

When my husband took my children, my mother came to where I was living and attempted to kill me also. Blood was running down my face from her hitting me in the head with a glass ashtray, so that added to the trauma, plus a few more truly traumatic things that happened at the same time. I actually got partial amnesia from that horror, and could not remember anything about my children except for my daughter, and her just a tiny bit. My sons still do not recognize me as their mother because they were all so young. I had made many suicide attempts from the age of ten through my life. I guess that was enough to confirm the diagnosis.

No tests were ever run to confirm my diagnosis, but I was given medication anyway. I am seventy-two now and fine, but that was how they handled mental illness when I was in my twenties and thirties. Many of the counselors I saw could not even deal with the things I had been through, so they kept turning me over to psychiatrists, who always just immediately ordered medications. I was never told anything about the relationship between my mental state and the proposed medication, and I was given just about every kind of medication over time you can think of—all those big names—Prozac, lithium, Zoloft, you name it. I had no idea what they were for except that I was told I was just depressed. I think I was a lot more than that.

The medication was truly a nightmare. I was walking stiff legged and like a zombie. They didn't even check me regularly to see how the medication was doing. They just kept giving me more and more. If I said I didn't feel well, they would just switch medications. I felt physically as though I was dead, and the depression did not go away. In fact, as time went on I became more and more withdrawn and unable to cope with just about anything.

The medicine I got when I was younger caused me to have kidney problems, and one doctor told me I was going to die from kidney problems. I thought, "Not," even as sick as I was, and I dumped all my meds down the toilet. My last suicide attempt was in the 1990s. It was so bad that I couldn't speak for about a week. I could hear what was being said but could not form words. I took pills, and the nurse was supposed to continue to pump my stomach, but quit too soon, so I did suffer from the medications.

I would have liked to been told more about all of those medications. I am extremely sensitive to medications and have many allergies from them and severe reactions. Once I was given Lyrica, and I got such horrible vertigo and sickness from it, I was hospitalized for a day or more. On balance, my experience with medications has been extremely negative. It honestly could have killed me because I feel now it was as if they were just experimenting on me.

What really helped me was when I got a counselor who really had been through things in his own life, and he was able to talk to me and help me think about things that had happened in my life. I always trusted him, and he gave me a lot of positive encouragement and was very kind. He listened to me as I cried so many tears, screamed at God, and generally went through the things that people go through when they are trying to get well. I think if I had not found someone so kind and understanding, and had not worked on forgiveness and other things, I would have never had a chance to get well.

I don't believe in medications for mental illness unless it is so severe that the patient will do harm to others or to himself or herself. These medications just hide the real problems and actually keep the patient from getting well again. Today, finally as an old lady, I have gotten well. Now I am seventy-two, have four volunteer jobs, one pretty major; I have had good careers, and currently work as a substitute instructional aide for special needs/emotionally disturbed children and have been doing that for about eight years.

I am much in demand. I have started a nonprofit to assist physically challenged artists, and we have had many, many exhibits to help them get exposure for their work. I joined a church I like very much and go regularly, and I am enrolled in a Christian university online back east, and am getting a second degree in paralegal studies. So life is full and good. It isn't easy sometimes. I have been severely bullied by other seniors in both mobile home parks I have lived in, even to the point of some other women trying to assault me. But I have gotten through it, and without any medications either. I will never take those kinds of medications again—any of them. Life is good and getting better by the day. I am really looking forward to the next ten years and beyond!

Jules

My first encounter with psych drugs was in the early 1980s. I was seeing a psychiatrist to help me through some rough transitions. My living situation was very difficult, and there came a day when I felt unable to uncurl from a chair in my bedroom. By the end of that day, I was very frightened about my condition and phoned the doc. I asked him if the next step was to check into a psych ward; he told me that was a "court of last resort" and that there were medications I could take. They weren't happy pills; they were to give me a chance to bounce up if I found myself way down.

When I met with him and received instructions on the meds (I don't know what they were, but shall we assume some kind of tricyclic?), he told me that I would need to stay on the meds for nine months, as this was the typical length of time that my body chemistry was in an altered condition. I felt helpless and put all my trust in the doc. The meds had powerful side effects—I don't recall their exact nature, though—but they did seem to do what they promised: they seemed to make it possible for me to spend only a very little time in the depths before I was able to bounce back up to a functional state. At least one side effect remained with me for decades: I had an almost constantly red nose.

Fast forward to 1991. Again, I was in a very difficult situation and felt unable to do anything reasonable to make changes. I burst into tears at the dinner table, had suicidal ideation, and so on. Fortunately, there had been some advances in the field, and I was put on one of the newer drugs. There were very few side effects, and I had a newfound resiliency for some six months.

A few years later, I heard a radio program in which people with chronic low-grade depression were interviewed. I recognized myself! Since puberty, I had been talking myself into getting out of bed nearly every day of my life. I began taking Wellbutrin with a side order of Prozac, and this combo seemed to work wonders for me for years. I really felt very grateful not to be slogging through my life as if the ground were gumbo.

However, hitting another circumstantial rough spot in 2005, I was having a lot of anxiety and wondered if my meds had stopped working for me. Thus began a period of a few years during which I went through various combinations of anti-depressants, then was re-diagnosed as bipolar, tried combos of drugs targeted toward that malady, and ultimately ended up back where I started, with something like dysthymia and a history of two clinical depressions. For the last several years, I've been taking Lexapro.

As things stand, I am looking forward to working with my current doctor (not a psychiatrist) to wean me off prescription anti-depressants through the use of acupuncture and herbs. I don't enjoy the current side effects of being nearly unable to cry and having a lowered sex drive. I also wonder what other things I might be missing in my life. As an artist, I need access to powerful feelings and experiences.

I sometimes consider a hypothetical trade-off situation: If going off the drugs meant a return to my former vulnerabilities but the loss of those side effects, which would I choose? I've learned a lot over the years, I have a lot of resources up my sleeve, but I find the blues a most elusive, difficult adversary. If it comes to it, I will probably have to choose the drugs. I will soon get to find out.

Jeanette

In my late twenties, I was working two jobs, dealing with marriage and family difficulties, and frustrated at the lack of progress in my writing life. I finally recognized that I might be experiencing depression when I had a few glasses of wine with dinner one night and noticed how much better I felt. The dread, anxiety, struggle, and lack of focus that I'd been tolerating for months briefly lifted, and I realized something was not right.

I was familiar with the symptoms because my mother had dealt with depression for years and was taking antidepressants to treat it. So I knew about the anhedonia, negative thoughts, and hopelessness. I just didn't realize that I might be depressed because I was still functioning, going to work, and meeting my commitments. When I realized I was depressed, I felt even worse, like a failure for having succumbed to depression.

I spoke to a psychologist friend that day, and she recommended that I see my GP. My doctor was able to see me within a few days. Given my family history of depression and my previous experiences (I had seen another doctor for depression several years earlier, but didn't take meds then), she was receptive to my concerns. She gave me a questionnaire that asked about my mood, thoughts, eating and sleeping habits, and based on that she determined that I did have depression. She prescribed the same antidepressant that was effective for my mother (Celexa).

I knew something of how SSRIs worked, and I understood that while the medication would help improve my mood and functioning, I also needed to begin therapy to support me in making changes to my life and thinking so that the underlying causes of the depression would be dealt with. I don't remember now exactly where this knowledge came from—my psychologist friend, my mother's experience, discussions with other therapists, online reading. I also knew that some people could never go off medication (i.e., my mother) while others might recover enough to manage their mental health without it. I didn't have any moral judgments about using medication, I just saw it as a tool that could help support my recovery.

The Celexa began working within a few weeks, and the relief was very welcome. It was like having shackles removed or having a windshield obscured by mud suddenly cleared. The cruel chatter in my head quieted down noticeably. This made it much easier to do the work of therapy with a clearer perspective on my life and choices. My initiative returned, as well as my ability to enjoy the pleasures of food, books, and friends.

I stayed on the medication for three years and then slowly began weaning off it with my doctor's supervision. I did have the brain flashes that can be a symptom of withdrawal, and they were mildly worrying, but they abated and eventually disappeared. Without the medication, I noticed a return of the depressive thoughts and mood, and for a time I was worried that I would slip back into the illness, but I continued with therapy and prioritizing my writing work, and was able to get to a place where I felt fully mentally healthy and strong.

I probably had a higher-than-usual understanding of the illness and medication because of my family experience and the extra reading I did. I was grateful that I was able to start and stay on a medication that was effective with minimal side effects. For me, antidepressants were definitely a positive experience. I'm really happy with the choices I made and the support I received, and I have no regrets.

Tina

I was diagnosed with depression when I was around thirty-one. I knew something was wrong even when I was around thirteen. I thought it was my situation: being a teenager, moving around a lot, PMS, etc. My doctor at the time gave me a questionnaire that I filled out, and I was diagnosed with moderate depression. I started off on Paxil. The side effects made me sleepy. I didn't feel sad, but didn't feel like doing anything, like going out.

My doctor then switched me to Effexor. It was basically the same. I noticed I didn't really care about anything, but it was OK. I was fine with that. I also noticed that my range of emotions was limited. Before I felt happy at times, sad at times, but now everything was OK. Fine. That was my only emotion. I told my doctor again that I was feeling apathetic and she switched me to Lexapro. I didn't feel like myself and just felt "numb."

I was on antidepressants for over four years and would not recommend it to anyone. I decided to gradually decrease my dose and safely stop taking them. My doctor never asked me if I wanted to do this, but

I think they are trained to keep people on them because big pharma keeps making money. It is not the answer. I saw a documentary where they gave a depressed girl mega doses of vitamin B6. Over time she improved, but doctors didn't think it was safe . . .

If I hadn't decided to get off those drugs, my doctor would have me on them today. A good doctor should only keep someone on them for a year. I understand more about the medical industry now and believe in being my own advocate for good health. I eat better, exercise, and find natural alternatives to any problems I have. Doctors can only help so much.

After I stopped my medication, I had all these images in my head . . . there were so many. It was like a switch was turned on. I never felt creative when I was taking medications. It was difficult to write or paint. I'm a graphic designer, so I rely on my imagination for my job. There definitely was a connection there. I'm so glad to be off of medications and back to my old self again.

Rachel

Oh, if only SSRI's had existed in the early seventies! I'm not certain, of course, but I suspect that a good dose of Prozac, or one of them, would have cracked my major depression. But then, who really knows. The meds I tried then (e.g., Elavil and Disipramine) had side effects and took too long to work; I didn't stay on either for very long.

For me, a major point is that the SSRI's never would have helped me in any way if I hadn't encountered a psychiatrist who was willing to work with dosing. I say this because more than once over the years I was started on SSRI's, including Paxil and Prozac, and because of starting at the recommended starting dose, which was too high for me, I couldn't tolerate how badly I felt and ultimately stopped taking the med.

I've seen it with other people, too. The starting dose put me, and them, into a zombified state. I didn't feel or talk right. The doctor insisted, "This will go away once you get used to it," but for someone already feeling poorly and not like themselves, having this last vestige of feeling in control of oneself taken away was not helpful. I know that many people give up on the meds quickly because of this.

When I finally did start and stay on Prozac, it was because the doctor took heed of what I told him and actually prescribed liquid Prozac so we could titrate the dosage up from a starting amount that was way smaller than any pill or capsule that was available. So over a period of several months the dosage was titrated up until it reached 10 mg., at which time I switched over to a pill.

At that time I was adamant about wanting to be on Prozac, not so much for depression but more for social anxieties I was experiencing, mainly, getting a panic response when I had to speak in front of groups. But then, the Prozac didn't help with this as much as I would have liked. At other times I had used a beta-blocker (Propanalol) for this purpose and that worked better at stopping the physical symptoms such as trembling, sweating and dry mouth.

I remain on Fluoxetine (Prozac) to this day, but I often consider getting off of it. Why? Because I suppose the drug does what it's supposed to (i.e., I don't get seriously depressed), but then I rarely feel extremely joyful either. The drug seems to have leveled me out into a basic stability that precludes strong mood swings in either direction. But that, I guess, is the goal, eh?

Sharon

I have been diagnosed with mild depression ever since age sixteen (I'm forty-seven now), with two distinct episodes of severe clinical depression. I was tried on every antidepressant known during the 1990s and was the most suicidal I've ever been in 1996. In the 1990s, at the urging of a family member who thought I had bipolar disorder, I had a complete two-and-a-half-hour psychiatric evaluation, and the only findings were that I likely had seasonal depression or seasonal affective disorder.

2003–2007 was the most traumatic period of my life that led me to what I believe is my current mission today, which I'll describe in a moment. Not only did I experience a cancer diagnosis and the subsequent treatment of my only young child, but I also experienced domestic violence with her father at the same time. In 2006, I was diagnosed by a psychologist with PTSD, or at least PTSS (posttraumatic stress symptoms)—I got the diagnosis simply by filling out a few depression and PTSD questionnaires and speaking to the psychologist for a bit.

Actually, I diagnosed myself first. After seeking several therapists, I finally found one who did work most aligned with healing for me personally. This involved some tapping, some visualization, some guided meditation bringing a compassionate figure into the trauma episodes, some talk therapy, and affirming/discussing my use of intuition and spiritual guidance.

I spent five years completely off medication from 2008–2012 and experienced all the warning signs of severe depression again in the winter of 2012. So I was put back on an antidepressant (Celexa) at the lowest dose possible (10 mg.) for a year. In 2013, I took a year of eco-psychology classes and I felt profound healing occur. I weaned myself off medication again and began what is now my life's work. My vision is to interrupt trauma stress of caregivers in hospitals by facilitating stress reduction, grounding and reconnection with nature.

For several years I have held onto my vision to create a movement across hospitals in the US and taken baby steps by creating a webpage, a blog, a Facebook page, and bringing my own nature images and sounds to people indoors, with zero funding while being a single parent who has worked at times sixty hours/week at a desk job to meet basic bills (I no longer work overtime for my mental health).

I have learned that some type of mindfulness practice, a committed daily meditation practice replacing TV, and nature connection are the top three forms of mental distress healing that truly work wonders!

Jennifer

I received the diagnosis of "manic depressive" (now bipolar) in my early twenties. (I'm now sixty-four). I accepted it after a time, then denied it, fought against it, tried to "cure it," then learned to live with it. No tests were run to confirm the diagnosis. However, last year when I read a book on bipolar disorder, it cited an article on brain imaging technology, such as magnetic resonance imaging (MRI), revealing the differences in the brains of bipolar people from the brains of people without the disorder.

I got my doctor (family physician) to order an MRI. I got a copy and was going to send it to the people doing the study, and then I found out from my psychiatrist I had received the wrong type of MRI, and the type that I needed would cost thousands of dollars and my insurance would not cover it. So I decided it was not worth it to find out something I already knew.

Many psychiatrists, psychologists, and general MDs have told me for the past forty years that I need to be on medication the rest of my life. However, none of them agreed on the medication I needed. In my thirties and forties, I was stabilized on lithium (only becoming depressed after bouts of physical illness, like pneumonia). When I was fifty, I took myself off lithium gradually because I thought I could control my depression with a new meditation practice. Four months later, I went into a deep suicidal depression that lasted for several months.

For the next thirteen years I would have stable months, then depression for months, followed by a few days of manic highs, then stability for a few months until the depression returned. I had many doctors who prescribed just about every antidepressant, anti-anxiety medication, mood-stabilizing drug and anti-convulsion drug available. A partial listing of the drugs I have been given since my twenties are as follows: Pristiq, Seroquel, Cymbalta, Ativan, Ambien, Zyprexa, Wellbutrin, Depakote, Paxil, Trileptal, Lithium Carbonate, Klonopin, Lamictal, Zoloft, Depakote, Tegretol, Prozac, Clozapine, Haldol, and Thorizine.

With the exception of lithium, none of those drugs ever worked for me, they only gave me terrible side effects. The last antidepressant I tried that brought me out of a deep suicidal depression (the only one that ever did) was Viibryd. It actually worked but put me into a manic high. I went off it. My doctor said if I ever got depressed again, just take some more, but start out in a low dose. I am now off medication, and I control my mental states with exercise, meditation, good nutrition and the right supplements, sleep, and talk therapy with a psychologist who has helped me to recognize what triggers my depression.

The things that I would have liked to know back then—and I did ask my doctors about them—they did not know the answers to. Medication in the field of psychiatry is still a place where there are more questions than answers and very few "known results." Doctors appear to be still in the experimental phase with a very long way to go in understanding how and why medication works, or doesn't work, with various patients.

My experience with drugs has been, for the most part, negative, the exceptions being lithium (however there were side effects and monthly blood testing for twenty years) and Viibryd (except for the uncontrollable manic high). The most negative thing is that I felt I was a game of Russian roulette for my doctors. They really didn't know what would work, what combination, what dose and what the outcome would be. It was always, "Let's give it sixty days and see what happens." When you are thinking of suicide every morning when you wake up, sixty days is an eternity.

9

On Cause and Effect

What causes all this pain and distress?

Wouldn't we like to know what "causes" our thoughts, feelings, and psychological experiences? What "causes" our behaviors, opinions, and personality? What "causes" our current state of mind and our view of the world? What "causes" us to be sad or happy, anxious or calm, pessimistic or optimistic? Wouldn't that be useful information, both for ourselves and for anyone trying to help us? Could anything be more useful to know . . . and, unfortunately, less possible to know? Isn't it likely that we may gain a better understanding of the nature of the universe than the causes of one human thought or feeling? We would love to know what causes all things human—but can we ever know?

First of all, what do we mean by "cause and effect"? Cause and effect are far from simple concepts. What's the difference between a cause, a factor, an influence, and so on? When is a single cause necessary and sufficient to create a certain effect? In classical philosophy the subject is usually taught by beginning with Descartes' example of one billiard ball striking a second billiard ball. The first billiard ball "causes" the second billiard ball to move. This might be thought of as the strict or simple sense of "cause and effect." In this example one thing is clearly linked to another thing in a logical, proximate, and seemingly singular and sufficient way.

However this sort of explanation never tells the whole story, since it is always possible to raise the question, "But isn't whatever caused the first ball to move the *real* reason that the second ball moved?" Indeed, you could wend your way back to the big bang and beyond in what is called infinite regression. Second, is this cause really sufficient for this effect to happen? What if the second ball were glued to the table? The first ball caused the second ball to move only because the second ball was free to move. Still, despite these many technical difficulties, this is what we most often mean by cause and effect: that one thing logically, proximately, singularly, and sufficiently caused another thing to happen.

A reasonable example of "strict causation" might be little Bobby falling out of a tree and breaking his arm. The fall caused the break. This appears straightforward enough. But the simplicity of this picture vanishes the instant we decide to focus our attention one place or another. We can identify multiple causes of anything just by virtue of the direction of our gaze, the nature of our questions, and the categories that we decide to create and include, and this is abundantly true with little Bobby and his fall.

If I ask you, "What caused Bobby's broken arm?" you might reply in any of the following ways, all of which imply one or another spin on cause and effect: "He's a reckless rascal," "Being a boy," "Fury at our divorce," "The ground," "Bad luck," or "Gravity." In addition, if you are playing the current illegitimate mental disorder naming game that I've described previously, you might also include "attention deficit hyperactivity disorder" or "childhood depression." Each of these is a different explanation as to what really caused Bobby's broken arm.

How you choose to look at the matter may have great consequences for little Bobby. If you go with "bad luck," Bobby may have full permission to keep climbing trees. If, however, you go with "reckless rascal," you might punish Bobby and curb his tree-climbing exploits. If you go with one of the mental disorder labels, you might agree to have Bobby put on one or more powerful chemicals. These differences matter to Bobby. In the first case we have a Bobby who is free to keep climbing trees, in the second case we have a restricted Bobby who may pine for climbing and grow distressed at his lack of freedom, and in the third case we've created little patient Bobby with a mental disorder label and a regimen of powerful chemicals with powerful side effects.

Then there's the important matter of what effect you choose to look at. You might treat the fall as the effect of interest—the broken arm might grab your attention. But you might instead find it more telling to examine what happened after the fall. If you do that then the fall becomes a cause, not an effect, and it is what happens next that is the attention grabber. Why was Bobby afraid to tell his parents about his broken arm? Why did no one take Bobby to the doctor until the next day? Why is Bobby blaming himself for what was probably an accident? By asking questions of this sort you announce where your interests lie. The broken arm you chalk up to gravity; it is what happens next that interests you.

The next complication is that an effect is also a cause and a cause is also an effect. Say that you hate your job, and that produces distress.

That distress is an effect. But that distress, existing as pestering thoughts, ambient anxiety, hormonal activity, and so on, affects your system and causes everything from insomnia to stomachaches. The distress is an effect of your job situation and also a cause of your insomnia. Of course, "ultimately" what is causing both the distress and the insomnia is the fact that you hate your job: but still in this chain of cause and effect, and in every causal chain, effects are causes and causes are effects. If we try to separate out "things that are causes" and "things that are effects" we will have oversimplified the matter and hurt our chances of understanding the complicated nature of causal chains in human affairs.

Who knows what the "real" or "ultimate" cause is of anything human? For example, the "real" cause of your fear of dogs may trace all the way back to an actual incident with a dog in childhood, a fear reinforced by all manner of "causes and effects" since then. Now each encounter with a dog "causes" you to panic. However, it is not so much the current dog barking at you that is the "real" cause of your terror but your experience with that "first" dog. But is that even right? Why did that first dog frighten you? Was there already something in your original personality primed to react negatively to a barking dog? Maybe the "real" cause is completely odd and oblique; maybe your fear has something to do with bared teeth, drool, or who-knows-what and not dogs at all. Who could ever say for sure?

I hope you can feel the tangle here and experience the first tendrils of overwhelm. You can see why, if I am tasked with helping you, I might be inclined to quickly offer you chemicals. You can see why I might invent some "most important thing to look at"—say, your dreams—so as to not have to look at all the rest. You can see why I might be inclined to repeat the incantation, "And how did that make you feel?" in lieu of knowing what else to say. You can see why I might accept your version of the story—say, that the pestering of your elderly mother is causing your current sadness—even though I suspect that your formed personality, which prevents you from entering into relationships or venturing out of the house, is the more real cause. All of these are infinitely easier ways to proceed than trying to discern what is "really" causing your distress.

In a medical or biological model, we have some reasonable ways of talking about cause and effect. A virus or a bacterium causes certain effects like fever and nausea. We then treat the cause, the virus or the bacterium, with one sort of medication. We may also treat the effects— the fever and the nausea—with other medications. In this model it is easy to talk about cause and effect, easy to understand how "symptoms of the illness" can be rightly considered effects that can be separately treated, easy to understand how the cause itself might be prevented and no longer troublesome to the species by virtue of, say, vaccines or water purification. While this is an oversimplification of how medicine actually works, it is not such a terrible distortion of the process.

Nothing like this can go on with mental health. We can dream of it going on—we can dream of finding the equivalent of infections that produce sadness and the equivalent of vaccines that will inoculate us against sadness—but that is a pipe dream. We can dream of finding the equivalent of bacteria that cause us to experience life as a cheat and the equivalent of medications that cure us of experiencing life as a cheat—but that is a pipe dream. You can see clearly why mental health professionals—unlike medical doctors who really must deal with the complications of cause and effect if they want to make accurate diagnoses—would want to wash their hands of cause and effect. Who wouldn't want to avoid this particular morass?

Let's put some additional difficulties on the table before we try to answer the question, "How should we proceed?" All of the following challenges confront us when we investigate how "cause and effect" operate in human affairs.

- The challenge of discerning differences in effects

  Is one sadness the same as another sadness? Are there differences among sorrow, grief, mourning, and despair? Can we discern differences in effects such as these that lead us to identify different causes? In medicine we regularly can. A certain sort of arm fracture suggests child abuse, and a different sort of arm fracture is congruent with falling out of a tree. Someone trained and experienced in these matters knows to look for these differences and can discern these differences. But in our sphere, and whatever her training, intuition, and wisdom, how good a job can a human experience specialist be expected to do in discerning some difference between, say, one expression of sadness and another? Given that there are no x-rays to take, no tests to run, and only questionable self-reports to go on, how refined a job can she be expected to do?

- The challenge of "idea as cause" and "idea as effect"

  For human beings, our thoughts, ideas, and opinions amount to powerful and singular causes and effects in our causal chains of distress. The idea of "cause and effect" in the physical world has about it the sense that one real thing is acting upon another real thing, like one billiard ball striking another billiard ball. But in human affairs, we have thinking to factor in. Consider all of the following. "I am having these troubles because of my bad deeds in another life." "The witch cursed me, and now I have these pains." "God is punishing me for my sins." Billions of people explain "cause and effect" in these ways. The "solutions" that naturally flow from these occult explanations of distress are charms, potions, prayers, incantations, offerings, and so on, solutions that are completely reasonable given the explanations at play. How do we deal with the fact that human causal chains include ideas?

- The challenge of describing an effect without inadvertently labeling the person

Let's say that you see some red dots on a person's arm. To instantly call those red dots "a rash" is already to characterize it and to hint at what you believe are its causes. But what if the dots are a tattoo? What if the dots have been painted on? What if he is a housepainter? In these three cases, calling those red dots "a rash" would amount to a fundamental mistake. You would be obliged to begin looking at "what causes a rash" or "how rashes are treated" when no rash is present. Likewise, if you shop a lot and I label you with a shopping addiction, I have set us up for "addiction work" just because of the language I've chosen to use. Can helpers train themselves to refrain from labeling and hone that surprisingly rare skill of observing without labeling? Can they witness sadness, mournfulness, gloominess, or despair and somehow prevent themselves from thinking "depression"? At the very least, can they grow better aware of the nature of this "inadvertent labeling" problem?

- The challenge of distinguishing a "cause" from a "factor," an "influence," and so on

In a strict sense, you can't cause me to strike you unless you wire me up to some apparatus that makes me involuntarily strike you. You can provoke me, influence me, affect me—but not cause me. Very often when we use the word "cause" in human affairs, we actually mean influence, affect, contribute, and so on. The one billiard ball causes the other billiard ball to move. What in life is like that? If I don't posit you with some free will not to strike me when I provoke you, if I conceptualize you as merely reflexive, determined, and robotic, haven't I done you some injustice? Likewise, if I imagine that some complex behavior on your part, something like marrying or divorcing, has been caused by some one thing, as opposed to arising from many influences and factors, aren't I terribly oversimplifying the matter? Do we ever actually mean "cause" in human affairs—or are we always talking about multiple factors, multiple influences, and so on?

- The challenge of factoring in the possibility of biological malfunction as a cause or the cause

As a human experience specialist, I would know that nothing of a biological nature has been proven to "cause" "effects" like "depression" or "schizophrenia." There are hypotheses galore regarding the biological "causes" of such "mental disorders"—but no proof and no compelling evidence. So would I want to send you for a workup when I already know that no tests exist to pinpoint any biological causes of "mental disorders"? On the other hand, if you have a thyroid problem that is causing your fatigue or a brain tumor that is causing your headaches, that is clearly another matter.

Given this complicated reality, that "mental disorders" are made-up labels but that there might still be something organic "causing" one or another of your "symptoms" or "effects," what is my best or most reasonable course of action? Might I create a handout that explains my views on biological cause and effect and that presents that a medical workup is imperative and yet may find nothing and may prove nothing? Would I offer up this conclusion not only to protect myself from litigation but also because this is what I believe, that in life some unwanted effects are of the biological malfunction sort while the vast majority are not?

- The challenge of the patent invisibility of most causes in human affairs

If you lash out at people because you feel cheated by life, how can I possibly comprehend that causal chain if, for example, you will not admit that you feel cheated by life and if you deflect all of my efforts at understanding your motives and your reality? What if a "root cause" of your anger is that you never got over the fact that you were adopted or that you were the product of rape and that information never gets on the table? Won't I be obliged to deal with the "effects," your anger and your lashing out, without having any access to the causal chain in play? You do not see cause and effect written in the look of graphite. You do not see the world of sub-atomic particles, the strong force holding nuclei together, or anything else about its history. If you did not know chemistry and physics you would know just about nothing about how cause and effect has operated to create the graphite in your pencil. Since we have nothing like chemistry or physics available to help us understand you, where does that leave us?

Simple Inquiry

Let's say that despite all of these challenges, a human experience specialist still wants to take a stab at understanding what is causing the distress a person is reporting. The way to proceed is actually simple and straightforward: ask. Yes, all that she would get is a self-report. But that self-report might be revealing. That human beings are regularly defensive and tricky doesn't mean that they aren't also sometimes truthful and insightful. Shouldn't we give them that opportunity? Shouldn't we give them the chance to help us—and help themselves?

What might this inquiry into cause and effect look like with someone who is willing to cooperate? It might amount to nothing fancier than filling out a questionnaire. The questionnaire, however, would have to allow breathing room for this complicated human being to have a chance to really think about the matter. Checking off boxes would not do. There would need to be space for long answers—which means that the information would then have to be read by another human being, not a machine. Clearly our human experience specialist would be making work for herself by virtue of her commitment to trying to understand.

What might such a questionnaire look like? Let's create a medium-sized one for the "presenting issue" of "despair." Let's hold it to thirty questions—it could easily be double that in length—and let's skip the details and explanations that would need to be included (for instance, we would need to define terms like "original personality" and "formed personality"). The following is the skeleton of what a full-fledged questionnaire might include:

1.   What is causing your despair?
2.   Have you despaired a lot in your life? If so, can you say why?
3.   Have you recently despaired more? If so, can you say why?
4.   What triggers your despair? Do you know?
5.   Has a particular incident triggered your despair? If so, do you know why that was triggering?
6.   Do you suspect some biological basis for your despair? What are your thoughts on that possibility?
7.   Do you suspect some psychological basis for your despair? What are your thoughts on that possibility? (Since this may prove the crux of the matter and since this may also prove too large and unwieldy a question to answer, try your hand at a bulleted list of 'psychological reasons for my despair.' Creating this bulleted list may help you identify many possible psychological sources or causes of your despair.)
8.   Are there historical reasons for your despair, events that have happened in your personal history?
9.   Are there dynamics or events from childhood that may have caused your despair?
10. Are there family dynamics that may have caused your despair?
11. What in your current circumstances might be contributing to or even causing your despair?
12. Looking at your work life specifically, is there anything about your work life that might be contributing to your despair?
13. Looking at your relationships specifically, is there anything about your relationships that might be contributing to your despair?
14. Do you have a strong sense of life purpose? If not, might that lack of life purpose be contributing to your despair?
15. Do you experience life as meaningful (or meaningful enough)? If not, might that lack be contributing to your despair?
16. Are you living your life aligned with your values? If not, might that be contributing to your despair?

17. Is there some important goal or dream that has eluded you and that continues to elude you? If so, might that be contributing to your despair?
18. Does your way of life suit you? If not, might that be contributing to your despair?
19. Are you happy with yourself? If not, might that be contributing to your despair?
20. Do you regularly make yourself proud by your efforts? If not, might that be contributing to your despair?
21. Is some strong emotion like rage simmering under the surface? If so, might that be contributing to your despair?
22. Do you have the sense that some features of your original personality are contributing to your despair?
23. Do you have the sense that some features of your formed personality—your worldview, your self-talk, your habits, the very "way that you are"—are contributing to your despair?
24. Is something about the culture in which you live contributing to your despair?
25. Is your physical health (or lack of physical health) contributing to your despair?
26. Are you currently under any special pressure? If so, do you suspect that is contributing to your despair?
27. Are you currently "out of control" in any way (for example, with your drinking, your eating, your sexual activity, etc.)? If so, is that lack of control contributing to your despair?
28. Has any recent random or stray thought triggered this despair?
29. Has any recent random or stray feeling triggered this despair?
30. What else might be contributing to your despair?

Would a filled-out questionnaire of this sort get a human experience specialist a full, true, or complete picture of cause and effect in this person's life? Probably it wouldn't. But would it provide interesting and useful information? I don't see how it could not. Even if the responses were scanty, defensive, evasive, rote, or anything else under the sun, even such responses would help her understand. As complicated as the concept of cause and effect is and as mysterious as the operations of cause and effect are in human affairs, this route of simple inquiry is bound to produce some useful dividends.

As a human experience specialist, you could go the route of formal inquiry with questionnaires and so on. You could also just guess. You might hazard a guess from what you've heard from the person sitting across from you and what you've observed about him. For example, it is not at all uncommon for a therapist to say something like, "Your father beating you may have made you very angry, and you may have squelched all that anger and become depressed instead of angry." The therapist is guessing (in the language of psychotherapy, "making an interpretation") about an unseen chain of causes and effects. This is a cornerstone interaction and technique of therapy.

The therapist is saying, "The anger is not visible to either of us, but my understanding of your story, human nature, and the look of your passivity suggest underlying anger to me." This "interpretation" may be extremely useful if the therapist has guessed right. But what if the therapist has guessed wrong? Then the relationship may in fact be harmed, as his client or patient (which is what he is calling the person sitting across from him) is now less likely to credit the therapist with insight. So guesses about cause and effect are double-edged swords, especially if they are presented too smugly and with too much conviction and assurance.

A human experience specialist would likewise sometimes guess but would use language to make it apparent. Displaying no conviction or assurance, a specialist might say, "I have absolutely no idea if the following is on point. But sometimes right underneath sadness is anger. Given your history of abuse, I could see that being true for you. Does that ring any bell for you?" There would be no hint of smug certainty, no reliance on the pseudo-science of theory, and no subtle or overt labeling. It's rather like a friend saying, "Are you maybe angry?" and completely different from a therapist saying (or rather thinking), "With this sort of neurotic passive-aggressive personality there's always anger just underneath the surface."

Cause and effect are the "Why?" "Why do you prefer frozen vegetables to fresh ones?" translates as "What is causing you to prefer frozen vegetables to fresh ones?" "Why are you drinking so much?" translates as "What is causing you to drink so much?" "Why do you stay at a job you hate?" translates as "What is causing you to stay at a job you hate?" In general, helpers respond to cause and effect in one of three ways. They inquire: that is the method and rationale of psychotherapy. They ignore: that is the method if not the rationale of psychiatry. Or they proceed directly to help: that is the method and rationale of coaching.

Since it is possible to proceed with the helping without investigating any cause-and-effect matters—AA works this way, for example, folding cause-and-effect questions into ideas like "powerlessness" and "disease" and moving right on to the tasks of sobriety—it is right if we ask, "Do we actually need to know much (or anything) about cause and effect in order to be of help?" Could a human experience specialist, rather like a coach, move right on to the present and the future without inquiring about possible causal chains that landed the person across from her in his current situation? Is that a legitimate option? We'll return to this question when we look at "what actually helps."

However, while it may prove possible for an individual sufferer or an individual helper to skip investigating cause and effect and move right on to the help, it is imperative that researchers do not. To the extent that we throw in the towel in the face of too much complexity, a terrible paucity of genuine knowledge, and what looks to be the very real possibility that we can't answer the questions we pose, to that extent we have allowed psychiatry and the chemical industry to win the battle over what constitutes "treatment" for distress. If research throws in the towel, if our best and our brightest avoid tackling the biggest questions of human nature and instead proceed down the narrow paths dictated by their academic discipline, then the future of mental health will remain firmly in the hands of chemical companies.

You may not need to know what is causing your sadness—it is possible that what you need to know is how to relieve your distress, not what has caused it. As a helper, you may not need to know what is causing the person across from you to be experiencing so much distress—it is possible that all you need to know is how to relieve that distress. But as a society, we need more. As a society, we desperately need a large-scale, focused inquiry into the mechanics of cause and effect in human affairs. As messy, unwieldy, frustrating, and even impossible an inquiry as that may prove to be, a future that includes better mental health depends on it.

10

Life Purpose, Meaning, and Value

It has become customary in the world of mental health services provision to call "mental disorders" biopsychosocial things. This way of characterizing made-up disorders has arisen for a number of reasons, the primary one of which is that biopsychosocial sounds like it is saying a lot when of course it is saying nothing in particular. As weak as it is, however, it is made even weaker by its explicit exclusion of distress arising for existential reasons. You mean to say that meaning, value, and life purpose count for nothing?

Providers of mental health services tend not to take a client's meaning needs, life purpose concerns, or conflicts of values into account. How often do you suppose a client is asked, "Tell me a little bit about your life purpose choices and decisions" or "Are you more a meaning-maker or more a meaning-seeker?" The answer is virtually never. These sorts of questions are not part of the everyday landscape that mental health service providers inhabit. There are a few exceptions to this rule, for instance among some existential psychotherapists, but as a rule the question "What really matters to you?" is rarely asked.

Most psychiatrists, psychologists, psychotherapists, and other mental health service providers don't possess an interest in the meaning, purpose, and value of life. They don't train in these three concepts or provide a coherent set of ideas or even a working vocabulary that would allow them to chat with clients about these matters. Indeed, they may never have thought about meaning, purpose, or value themselves. Does the average mental health service provider have a clear understanding about the requirements to make meaning: what it takes to influence, create, and provoke the psychological experience of meaning? Have they thought through how people can be helped to name and frame their life purposes? Most surely have not.

Can it really be the case that it doesn't matter to a client whether or not he is living according to his values and principles or contrary to his values and principles? How mentally or emotionally healthy can a person be expected to feel if he is not making meaning and not manifesting his life purposes? If living bereft in those ways, don't we expect a person to feel sad and anxious, don't we suppose that he will be pulled in the direction of meaning substitutes and anxiety soothers? Why wouldn't a person be expected to fill up on sex or shopping or cookies or Scotch in the absence of meaning?

Nor is such a conversation so difficult to have. It is really not so hard to paint a picture of what value-based meaning making might look like, what it would feel like to make daily meaning investments and seize daily meaning opportunities, what it would take to create your own personal menu and mix of meaning opportunities, and what the process looks like for naming and framing your life purposes. The main problem seems to be that these matters are not on the radar of mental health service providers. They are fixated on the current model of "diagnosing and treating mental disorders," a discredited labeling model that ought to be jettisoned as quickly as possible.

To be sure, their training programs fail them—almost certainly they have never taken a single class in which meaning or life purpose was discussed. Their leaders are failing them too, as virtually all of them have ties to the pharmaceutical industry and our current pill-pushing mentality. Nor are clients themselves helping much, as they have gotten into the habit of presenting their difficulties in terms of sadness, anxiety, addictive behaviors, and so on rather than as existential difficulties having to do with meaning and life purpose. If a client does not bring it up and his therapist likewise does not bring it up, how will it ever get on the table?

If we want our mental health service providers to do a better job of realizing what actually matters to human beings, how life purpose and meaning issues are implicated in emotional distress, and what they as providers can do to help, there are a minimum of four steps to take in that direction:

1. Providers must come to their own personal understanding of the value of discussing meaning and life purpose with clients. Do they sincerely believe that issues of meaning and life purpose aren't important? They must come around to valuing the importance of meaning and life purpose in human affairs and, having made that pivotal change in

outlook, demand of themselves that they include life purpose, meaning, and value in their conversations with clients.

2. Providers must arrive at some concepts about meaning and life purpose that they themselves believe and understand. If you yourself have no idea where meaning resides, how a conflict in values can be resolved, what it takes to make a strong life purpose decision and then stand behind that life purpose decision, and so on, how helpful can you be in helping others make meaning and live their life purposes?

3. Providers must adopt or create language that allows them to talk intelligently with clients about life purpose, meaning, and value. This idiosyncratic language might sound like, "Let me tell you what I mean by a meaning investment and why that might be important for us to talk about" or "There's a practice I'd like to tell you about called a morning meaning check-in that might help you orient your day around your meaning intentions." Without such a vocabulary in place, conversations about meaning and life purpose are nearly impossible.

4. Providers must be willing to bring these matters up with clients if clients do not bring them up themselves. By bringing these matters up they will be better able to tackle what is causing their client's distress, rather than circling around the "symptom picture" of what the distress looks like. The likelihood may be great that, for example, your client's sadness is neither biological nor psychological in nature but existential instead. Wouldn't that be important to get at?

All of this is surprisingly easy to accomplish if only mental health providers took an interest. Consider the following example. Here is the complete email exchange between a young man we'll call Michael, who wrote me out of the blue, and me. Michael wrote:

Dear Dr. Maisel,

I have been going through a hard time for as long as I can remember and have pursued every option available to me without feeling like I've gotten 'better.' I am twenty-seven and male. I was hoping you could give me some advice about what course of action I might take next. I am going to try to make this email brief as I have a tendency to go on and on when talking about this subject.

My mental health history is long and complex so I'll summarize by saying I was diagnosed with ADHD as a kid and took Ritalin until around the age of eleven. I was then diagnosed with depression and anxiety and placed on Paxil, which gave me the symptoms of bipolar disorder that I was subsequently diagnosed with and for which I was treated for years. All of these treatments made me increasingly sick and unmotivated.

I finally went off all medication before I started college (around age eighteen), and eventually ended up at a university where I studied and had a decent time other than a couple of serious life crises and occasional bouts of depression and anxiety. I graduated with highest honors and a very good GPA, but by the time I graduated I was beginning a depressed episode that would be nearly continuous from the age of twenty-two until the present. I started smoking marijuana to cope with severe anxiety and depression around that time and have done so on and off since then.

I worked two very different jobs in very different places, both provoking extreme anxiety, boredom, isolation, and frustration in me, although my coworkers and management all liked me and were upset when I decided to leave. Now, I am living with my father in a very rural community where I am more isolated than ever, more anxious and more depressed than ever. I spend most of my time reading about depression, exercising and meditating when I feel like I can, and reading a lot of fiction and philosophy in addition to psychology.

I have almost no contact with the outside world other than occasional shallow conversation with neighbors (which I dread) and seeing my therapist once a week, but she isn't helpful and is mostly grounded in a form of Buddhist psychology I find very vacuous and unappealing. If I start talking about the meaning of life, she says things like 'But don't you want to be happy?' as if I'm being a jerk by worrying about something as insubstantial as "meaning."

Everything in life feels like a chore. There is nothing I can imagine doing for long enough to make money from it. Occasionally I will get extremely interested in a subject or project, which has always been the case throughout my life, but instead of lasting for months like these interests used to, I become disenchanted and bored within a day or at most a week. After that I can't even force myself to engage with that topic anymore without feeling severely depressed. I've tried to get a job but anxiety, aversion, disinterest and a sense of pointlessness just hammer me to the ground every time something comes up.

On top of all of that, or maybe at the core of it, is the fact that I just hate myself. I feel like I've squandered my life away and like I don't even deserve to feel better or have anything good from life because I have no talents, no skills, and nothing that makes me special other than this grinding depression. Most recently I travelled to a foreign country using some of the last of my savings, hoping for some kind of epiphany or change of heart. Instead I just felt incredibly alone and realized the emptiness even of beautiful beaches and the warm sun. It all just felt like it was being wasted on me, a piece of garbage with no hope for a decent life.

I'm contacting you because I've read parts of some of your books. I've tried to follow the programs in them but got stuck early on. I just kept getting overwhelmed by the pointlessness of it all and by my own lack of talent or anything particular to say. *Rethinking Depression* felt promising but I just haven't been able to come up with any meaning that could possibly apply to my own life. I have nothing to offer and I don't want anything particular from the world, so the obstacles I come up against immediately frustrate me to the point of complete apathy. I'm only writing this email because I'm desperate, but I have no idea what I'm desperate for. Maybe to feel like less of a loser and to think that maybe I'm worth something.

I don't know how to make this more coherent or tighten it up so I'll just leave it there. If you have any advice, thoughts, or can point me in some direction, I'd appreciate it. If you need more information please let me know as well. Thanks in advance.
Michael

To this I replied:
Hello, Michael:
Well, you are at a good age to make some new meaning investments ☺. As you probably know but perhaps need to remind yourself, you will have no life purposes until you choose your life purposes and little sense of meaningfulness until you make decisions about what meaning investments you want to make and what meaning opportunities you want to seize.

You ought not to expect life to "feel" meaningful—you have to dig into your values and principles and decide what sort of life would make you proud—that is, you must manifest your values and principles and, if you are lucky, experience life as meaningful as a result of having made those efforts. That's it in a tiny nutshell ☺. Good luck to you!
Best,
Eric

To my reply Michael wrote:
Thank you for the fast response. I know that there is no meaning unless I create it. But no matter how much I think about that and try

to execute it, any meaning I come up with feels as empty as anything else and doesn't motivate me to do anything differently.

For example, I came up with a meaning statement that was something like "I want to live in a way that I can feel proud of" a la Sartre. But my mind is still incredibly scattered and the words end up meaning nothing after a few days, when I try to think up a new meaning statement. I did this for a few weeks before finding I could no longer continue this cycle because it felt so hollow. I'm not sure what to do now.
Michael

To this I replied:

It isn't a life purpose statement that you need now—the one you articulated is just fine ☺. It is that you have to muster the energy and the inner resources to TRY some prospective meaning opportunities to see if they in fact pan out. Meaning opportunities come with no guarantees. They are absurd, optimistic, hopeful guesses about what might existentially work.

Volunteer for something, write something, relate to someone, start juggling in public, do something completely different, try something—basing your guesses on the values and the principles you want to uphold. Make your life count by TRYING something—only then will you be able to see if that something 'mattered enough.' Yes, you have tried this before—and you must try it again. Create a new list of meaning opportunities—that's step one. Then DO some of them—that's step two.
Best, Eric

Michael ended our brief correspondence with the following reply:

Thank you. I will give this a try. It actually helps a little to realize that there is no other option.

Does this amount to a complete examination of Michael's meaning needs and meaning realities? Of course it doesn't. Will this little interchange turn Michael's life around? Probably it won't. But isn't it interesting that Michael found even this minimal interaction helpful? What if a human experience specialist worked with Michael in the areas of value, life purpose and meaning? What if that—and not Michael's putative "mental disorders"—were the focus of the work? Isn't it just possible, bordering on quite likely, that such a focus would do more for Michael than more pills, new pills, or "therapeutic talk" about his upbringing?

The future of mental health requires that we add this focus and make it a priority. There is no reason why we can't begin to take a sophisticated view of the relationship between life purpose, meaning, and value, on the one hand, and distress relief, mental wellness, and physical wellness, on the other. In this sophisticated view, it will become better understood that human beings might want to exhaust themselves in the service of some life purpose and by so doing create distress and physical problems; yet at the same time, even as they create that distress and difficulty, they may be providing themselves with exactly what they need and even be creating "genetic happiness," that deep happiness that comes from living our life purposes, experiencing meaning, and expressing our values.

In this sophisticated view, it will be understood that both can be true, that living as a value-based meaning maker can hurt, but that it can also help. We will begin to accept—even honor—the distress that arises because we have decided to fight for some cause close to our heart, struggle with some mind-breaking scientific problem, or paint the ceiling of our Sistine Chapel. We will then work to reduce that distress, insofar as that is possible, without calling the cause of that distress, our meaning-making efforts, into question. We will never say, "Don't make meaning—it is causing you too much distress." Rather we will say, "What can we do to reduce your experience of distress even as you pursue your meaning-making efforts?"

We will also add, "And by the way, it may be that your genes love it that you are living your life purposes." In a report on Mother Nature Network on the work of Steven Cole and his team at UCLA, Melissa Breyer explained, "The researchers assessed and took blood samples from eighty healthy adults who were classified as having either hedonic or eudaimonic wellbeing. Hedonic wellbeing is defined as happiness gained from seeking pleasure; eudaimonic wellbeing is that gained by having a deep sense of purpose and meaning in life. The study showed that people who had high levels of eudaimonic wellbeing showed favorable profiles with low levels of inflammatory gene expression and exhibited a strong expression of antiviral and antibody genes. For the pleasure seekers, the opposite was true; those with high levels of hedonic wellbeing showed an adverse gene-expression profile, giving high inflammation and low antiviral/ antibody expression." Human experience specialists can begin to make the case that there may be an "invisible" upside to living our life purposes.

We might fancifully call this invisible upside "genetic happiness." A writer might struggle writing his novel and as far as he can tell writing it is making him sad and ill, so poorly is the novel going and so much work does it require. Yet his mental and physical health may be better than if he wasn't making the attempt. To continue our fanciful way of saying it, his genes may be singing and dancing, profoundly happy knowing that their host is living one of his life purposes. Maybe this is true and maybe this isn't, but isn't it worth considering and isn't it worth researching? What if our mental health really is contingent on us attempting the things we say that we value? Such attempts may not matter at all from some universal perspective but they may matter a great deal to the individual.

Human experience specialists, in addition to speaking in a language that promotes a focus on life purpose, meaning, and value, might also suggest all sorts of tactics that help the people they work with identify their life purposes, live their life purposes, create meaning, maintain meaning, and get their values and principles onto their daily to-do lists. I mentioned earlier that we need tactics rather than taxonomies, and nowhere is that need greater than in the areas of meaning and life purpose. The people we are serving do not need and can't make any use of abstract philosophical discussions. Instead, they need tactics and specifics.

For instance, a human experience specialist might suggest that people learn "the new habit of quick meaning repair." Every day we're bombarded by small and sometimes large threats to our experience of life as meaningful. Maybe you're a writer and get a particularly painful rejection. Suddenly writing and even life itself may seem that much less meaningful. Or maybe you've invested meaning in your home business. Just as you're about to launch your product, you notice that someone has beaten you to the punch. You're likely to experience that bit of bad luck as a blow to your sense of the meaningfulness of life. Here's where a new habit of quick meaning repair would come in supremely handy.

First, you recognize that something important has happened. You admit that an existential blow has occurred. Second, you feel the feeling. Emotional health isn't helped by denial. Third, you remind yourself that meaning, because it is a psychological experience, is a wellspring and a renewable resource and that you can make new meaning as soon as the pain subsides. Fourth, you actually make new meaning by taking appropriate action. You send out your novel again or you actively market your product despite the new competition.

When a meaning crisis occurs, we become emotionally unwell, usually calling the experience "depression." Rarely do we recognize that a negative meaning event has occurred and that, in order to feel better, we must take action by making new meaning. It is therefore highly useful to acquire this four-step habit: understand what's happened, feel the feeling, pledge to make new meaning, and make some new meaning. All of this a human experience specialist might teach. No need to invoke Hegel, Kierkegaard, Sartre, or Camus. By creating simple, sensible, effective tactics, a human experience specialist can prove of great help even in the elusive territories of meaning and life purpose.

Another simple tactic, one that a human experience specialist might teach, is to suggest that a person create a menu of meaning opportunities (having first explained what that phrase means); envision a day that includes some meaning opportunities along with life's other tasks, chores, and responsibilities; and then try to live such a day. As simple as this tactic is, it represents valuable, even life-changing work that people rarely attempt. Here is the report of a participant in one of my life purpose boot camp classes after spending a week with the above assignment.

"I have considered myself for quite some time to be a 'meaning' sort of person, that is, on a quest to find and live a meaningful life. But in thinking about meaning opportunities I began to realize that I had not deeply or practically considered what 'meaning' is or what it entails to live a meaningful life. My past efforts have very much been focused on a kind of heavy-handed 'making meaning,' often with inconsistent, disappointing, or confusing results. Shifting to 'an opportunity mindset' was huge for me. There was a wonderful feeling of relief. Not every attempt to 'find meaning' has to succeed! We have opportunities, and some may pan out, and others may not; and eliminating the sense of failure if meaning isn't experienced takes the pressure off from the get go.

"As I say, realizing that the menu includes opportunities as opposed to guarantees took the pressure off. I was then much more able to approach this exercise in a fun, curious and expansive way. When I first sat down, I started with general categories (spending time with family, watching a beautiful sunset, etc.). But as I was going about my day, I became mindful in a much more specific, practical way of moments occurring that were meaning opportunities. I also knew that the exercise was rumbling around somewhere in the background of my brain. I'd be driving or doing something else other than this exercise and all of a sudden a specific experience would pop into my brain and shout, 'that was a meaning opportunity!' I loved this!

"I also realized that much of my day is spent in nonmeaning opportunity things. I particularly struggle with shifting from the way of life I've lived until recently (a workaholic unfulfilled lawyer) to a new way of living a flourishing and meaningful life. At the bottom line, I hit the question of how do I make an income to support myself when the items on my meaning opportunities list seem mostly intangible (a heartfelt conversation with my son, belly rubs for my dog)? As I've struggled with this issue this week, one exciting alternative came to mind. I'm going to try to take my current period of unemployment as a super-large meaning opportunity to chart my next course and to pay real attention to the idea that we pick our own life purposes. By engaging with this simple exercise of 'creating a menu of meaning opportunities' I feel like I am getting closer to the underneath of things."

It is easy to paint a picture of a contemporary "meaningless" day. You wake up, get on your treadmill of obligations, get into traffic, spend an hour getting to a job that does nothing for you except pay the rent, spend eight or more hours there, get back into traffic, arrive home, fret about dinner, handle some more obligations like bills and family crises, and try to find a program on television that will take your mind off the fact that you have not lived any of your life purposes or made any meaning on that day. The reality of this sort of day demoralizes people everywhere, and the specter of it haunts young people who want something different but have no idea what that different life might look like.

Given these realities, it is clear why so many people opt for denial. Nevertheless, mental health service providers must not be afraid to face these client realities. Yes, there may look to be few good answers. Yes, this may go far beyond "diagnosing and treating" made-up mental disorders. Yes, this may take a provider into territory that he is not trained to navigate and which he may not be navigating that well himself. But to ignore his client's meaning and life purpose needs is preposterous and ignoble. Our human experience specialist of the future will go right there and say, "We have some really difficult things to look at, ready or not." Our specialist may not be ready, and the person sitting across from her may not be ready either, but the inquiry will nevertheless begin.

11

Setting the Bar

What can we expect from members of our species with respect to their own mental health? How free are they to shed the shackles of their formed personality? To what extent are they equal to tackling the hard things required of them to reduce their distress, tasks like leaving meaningless work and finding or creating meaningful work, getting a grip on their mind and aligning their thoughts with their intentions, maturely looking reality in the eye while heroically naming and living their life purpose choices, and so on. Are human beings free enough for this? Smart enough for this? Mature enough for this?

Where should we set the bar with respect to what we can reasonably expect of our fellow human beings? Should we set it fairly high, at some middling level, or really quite low? The experiments run by social scientists suggest that we had better set the bar quite low. The experiments of social psychology paint a picture of man as a thoughtless herd animal, as someone easily manipulated, carelessly sadistic, and adamantly unaware. Milgram's famous learning experiments, for example, exposed human beings as creatures willing to deliver electroshock to their fellow creatures for no other reason than being told that they should. Zimbardo's equally famous prison experiments showed us how quickly average college students became sadistic prison guards or weak, frightened prisoners in virtually a matter of moments.

In Asch's well-known conformity experiments, in which subjects were asked about the lengths of lines, fully 75 percent of subjects announced that one line was the same length as another line, even though it transparently wasn't, just because others in the room said that it was. In Darley and Batson's Good Samaritan experiment, seminary students on the way to deliver a lecture on the importance of being a Good Samaritan could not be bothered to stop and help a person in distress. These and scores of other revealing experiments prove that the majority of human beings, and sometimes virtually everyone in a given experiment, seem incapable of thinking for themselves, acting in accordance with their professed values, withstanding peer pressure and other social pressures, or keeping their shadowy—and often barbaric—instincts at bay.

Therefore why should we expect the average person to rise to the occasion and think clearly, courageously, and smartly about his mental health or dispute the current system of mental disorder labeling? As an unaware herd animal, if that is what each member of our species primarily is, why should he be expected to do anything but accept what putative experts tell him he should believe? If even graduate students in psychology are unable or unwilling to see through the charade presented to them in their abnormal psychology classes, why should we expect someone in distress who is accustomed to buying what his society is selling to stand up and object?

Imagine running the following experiment, one designed to see how easily subjects embraced some new "mental disorder" label and willingly began a regimen of chemicals to "treat their disorder." A doctor dressed in hospital garb comes in and explains that it has recently been discovered that boredom is a mental disorder. He would give it a fancy name and describe symptoms of the disorder, symptoms chosen because all human beings experience them on occasion. He would make up some number—say, 75 percent—and claim that 75 percent of Americans suffer from this mental disorder and that a new drug is now available to treat it. By the end of this experiment, how many people in the room would agree that they had this mental disorder and would begin taking this "medicine"?

Likely everyone, if previous studies on the thoughtlessness, susceptibility, and gullibility of human beings are any indication. It is a fair guess that a doctor dressed in hospital garb would be able to turn almost every subject into a "mental patient" with little or no effort. Would anyone raise an objection and exclaim, "Wait, boredom isn't a mental disorder! It's a natural reaction to something boring you! Maybe it means that you need to think through your relation to life to see if you've made strong enough life purposes choices—maybe it's a 'symptom' of a meaning problem—but you shouldn't take a chemical to cure yourself of a lack of life purpose! That's insane! What blather are you promoting here?"

Would even one person in the room rise to make that speech or to voice some similar objection? Odds are they wouldn't. Would it matter if the room were filled with Bolivians, Japanese, Germans, or Americans? Probably not, since the experiments of social psychology are often run across cultures with identical results. Would it matter if the group were all men or all women or a combination of both? That probably wouldn't matter either. In all cultures where medicine is respected, it's a fair bet that folks in that room would open their mouths wide and start a drug regimen for their newly diagnosed mental disorder.

Still, we have some indications that human beings may be better, smarter and stronger than this. Who, observing our self-interested species, would have ever predicted human rights, civil rights, democratic ideals, humanist values, or advocates for freedom? Those realities, even if they are only fragilely in place and the result of the efforts of only a handful of people, speak to the possibility that the bar is moveable.

If an individual finds himself in a milieu where human rights and civil rights are touted, isn't he that much more likely to buy those ideals and in the process add his voice to their success? Likewise, if he were to find himself in a milieu where he was invited to take charge of his mental health, consider the many options available to him to reduce his experience of distress, think maturely and realistically about the creature that he is, and find himself supported in the idea of value-based meaning making, might he not grow into a more adept mental health self-helper?

Could society, by promoting certain values and by suggesting certain tactics, actually help make individuals in that society freer to think for themselves, help themselves, and stand up for themselves? Can a given cultural climate increase an individual's capacity for thoughtful reflection and courageous action such that, when confronted by choices that test his values and his capacity to make himself proud, he announces that two lines of unequal length are indeed of unequal length or that he has no sufficient reason to administer electroshock to the person sitting on the other side of the glass? Wouldn't such a society-wide effort be worth a try?

Unfortunately, society is not only uninterested in making such efforts, it has powerful reasons to stand antagonistic to such efforts. Given that the vast majority of constituencies in a society—churches, corporations, politicians, advertisers, etc.—are invested in people not acting too freely, smartly, or bravely, why would society rise up to help? What would be their motivation to improve the individual? So we have a second reason to feel obliged to set the bar low: that society wants it set low. Given the nature of the species, with its penchant for thoughtless conformity, and the nature of the societies that we form, societies that promote obliviousness and thoughtlessness, we can't feel too optimistic about raising that low bar to some greater height.

Nature's Method is Our Madness

The conserving nature of personality itself is a third factor that forces us to picture the bar as set quite low. The conserving nature of personality fights against our ability to act freely and improve our mental health. Personality is both who we are and who we can be. It is our fixed nature and our freedom all rolled into one package, a package that can be conceptualized as more static, passive, and determined or more dynamic, active, and free depending on what light we want to shine on ourselves. Which conceptualization seems truer?

When we dynamically, actively, and freely go against our own grain and surprise ourselves by standing up when we are usually meek, entering into recovery when we want another drink, or sitting down to write our novel when previously we always fled the encounter, we look like one sort of creature. When instead we do not surprise ourselves, when we have that next drink, when we avoid the creative encounter, when we fail to stand up and say, "No!" we look like that other sort of creature, that static, passive, determined one.

So, are we more static or more dynamic, more passive or more active, more determined or more free? On balance it seems that nature has made us rather more static, passive, and determined—really by a long shot. It is a feature of nature that creatures remain themselves for the sake of their integrity. It would not be good for bears as a whole if each individual bear suddenly got it into its head to fly. It would not be good for beavers if each individual beaver no longer saw the use of dams. Nature does not see it as good for our species as a whole for human beings to easily override the habits they learn as they develop, since nature supposes—correctly enough, since we are still here—that locking in habits is a basic evolutionary good.

It might seem sensible if a creature like us could more easily "evolve" and make smart, useful changes in the direction of personal happiness or distress relief. It may be true that such an idea makes sense as far as the individual goes. But nature isn't interested in the individual. It isn't interested in anything. Rather, it is a certain dynamism producing one experiment after another and apparently this experiment—us—is built to experience personality as rather a straightjacket. We get quite stuck because stickiness is an evolutionary virtue.

That nature doesn't care about individuals explains a great deal about our difficulties. If it cared about individuals, who would smoke cigarettes and invite cancer? If it cared about individuals, who would be permitted to experience the kind of psychological pain that leads to suicide? Unfortunately, nature's method is our madness. The conserving nature of personality maintains our distress while maintaining our self. This is an artifact of evolution.

It would be excellent if we came with a release valve that allowed us to periodically shed the thoughts that don't serve us, the feelings that pain us, the habits that mire us, and everything else worth discarding. If we had that release valve, we might have perfect mental health. But we don't possess that brilliant convenience. We are built without an easy way to change, which is sensible enough from an evolutionary perspective but really tremendously unfortunate for each individual human being.

We could perhaps improve our species-wide mental health in a generation if we taught our children to face the fact that their own personality is more a problem to them than a blessing and that, because of this evolutionary reality, they must think long and hard about how to upgrade that personality, insofar as nature allows for such upgrading. We might say to each child, "You are a unique, wonderful human being," encouraging them to build a healthy sense of self, while at the same time warning them about their responsibility to become a person equal to life's challenges. This twin message would not be very hard to craft. It might sound as simple as, "Be you but also become you."

Because the conserving nature of personality maintains distress and because change is uncomfortable work, we should expect, for example, that a person who claims to want to be less sad will do surprisingly little to actually become less sad. This is exactly what we see. To take another example, we see only the tiniest percentage of anxious people learn any anxiety management techniques. In the model I've described elsewhere of personality being comprised of original personality, formed personality, and available personality, the conserving nature of original personality and the restricting nature of formed personality look to limit our available personality significantly.

It is odd to say that a person who is chronically sad remains chronically sad because of a creaturely inclination to conserve a formed sense of self—and yet that looks to be the case. It is easier to stay sad than become a different person. It is easier to repeat charges against the world than to stop bringing those charges. It is easier to fear the same thing over and over again, even when it has proven no threat, than to stop fearing it. It is an evolutionary feature of personality to stay sad, keep leveling those charges, and remain fearful of shadows, no matter how much pain we create for ourselves in the process, rather than become someone new.

When dinosaurs go extinct, their time is over. Nature can't replace them because nature can't make creatures out of whole cloth. Evolution is a process, not a delivery system for fully formed creatures. Likewise, it can't replace a creature like us, one that has evolved with the stickiness of personality that we consistently observe, with a new creature that is freer to change and better able to eliminate distress. That stickiness serves evolutionary purposes, not individual purposes, and each individual is stuck with that biological reality.

Also part of our inheritance, however, is our ability to recognize that we are stuck. We might actually be able to make great use of that ability if we ever decided to pay some real attention to it. If we decided to deal with the fact that nature's methods help produce our madness, we might instantly grow up a bit and better face what nature has handed us.

Executive Awareness

How can we recognize that we are stuck if we are stuck? Well, human beings sometimes can, though whether the mechanism that allows them to step back and act more freely is a hugely complicated one or a radically simple one is completely unknown at the moment. Let's opt for simplicity and imagine that there is some single mechanism that allows a person to "be as free as one can be."

Imagine that you had the ability to snap your fingers and create enough distance between whatever you are thinking, feeling, doing, and experiencing to allow for thoughtful reflection. Even if you were at the height of a compulsion—say, to drink, to join a gathering mob, or to spend extra time at your job against your better judgment—you could nevertheless snap your fingers and inquire of yourself, "Should I have this drink?" "Should I join this mob?" or "Should I really keep working?" By snapping your fingers, you would provide yourself with the opportunity to be smart and sensible.

Picture that for a moment. Let's call this skill, ability, mindset, or personality trait "executive awareness." Let's suppose that this executive awareness is some mix of conscience, ego, rationality, thoughtfulness, and so on. We don't need to define executive awareness too carefully, as it is just a metaphor. But it may prove a useful metaphor since it is one possible way of conceptualizing two things: what human freedom might look like and what a person might hold as a personal mental health goal.

Isn't the essence of what we mean by both human freedom and mental health that an individual has the "space" in which to make a thoughtful choice? By obtaining that space, a person has the chance to, say, not administer electroshock to a stranger for no good reason or not agree that two lines of different lengths are the same length. Isn't it this "space" that allows us to refrain from having an affair that ruins our marriage, volunteer to fight in a war waged for shadowy motives, or stay locked in our sadness? Isn't this "space" both a breath of fresh air, one that allows the mustiness in our mind to dissipate, and also an opportunity to do the next right thing? Picture a skill, ability, or mechanism of this sort and ask, "Wouldn't it be nice to have that?"

Anything that helps a person step back from the causal chain, the complicated chains of cause and effect discussed in the last chapter, and apply thoughtfulness to a situation must be counted as a boost to freedom. The opposite would be impulsivity, lack of insight, rigidity, straightjacketed personality, thoughtlessness, and so on. Even if that "stepping back" is itself caused, as of course it must be, isn't that felt sense of freedom and the consequences of that felt sense of freedom—consequences like mindful choosing, value-based meaning-making, heightened executive awareness, etc.—so vital to mental health that we ought to come down on the side of promoting it?

Indeed, we might go a step further and assert that "mental health" is in essence a certain sort of self-relationship, a self-relationship of genuine overseeing. An inability to step back keeps us close to and embroiled in the distress. When we can't step back and employ our executive awareness, there is no distance between our selves and our stress, our painful feelings, our pestering thoughts, our rage, our despair. We are stuck, glued to the distress. In this regard, the cultivation of executive awareness might help across the board with regard to every so-called mental disorder.

Say that a person is plagued by that combination of appetite, raw energy, desire, meaning crisis, pestering self-talk, and racing brain pressure that we nowadays label as "mania." Little seems to help with this affliction except, as a band-aide of a home remedy, hot showers, and as a more dramatic intervention, chemicals. But what if increased executive awareness served both as a preventative, allowing an individual the chance to employ some method to dispute the mania, and as an intervention in the moment, allowing just enough space to keep the mania mediated rather than unmediated? We do not know if this is possible because we do not promote the cultivation of this ability to step back. Who knows if "increased executive awareness" might not eliminate "full-blown mania"?

Consider a second example. Let's take something that a person looks never to be able to fully get over and which might produce lifelong sadness or a lifelong background coloration of sadness. Let's say that a mother let go of her child's hand for an instant and that child ran into the street, was hit by a car, and was killed. It is easy to imagine that mother never getting over her grief and guilt. While we do not know, cannot know, and will never know why one woman in that set of circumstances manages to live a good life despite her recurring or constant pain and another mother falls apart and, say, is constantly "clinically depressed," becomes an alcoholic, or commits suicide, it is not hard to imagine that one crucial difference might be a capacity for executive awareness.

Who knows if this makes sense? But it is at least suggestive of the ways that we might think of "raising the bar" with any given human being. As a human experience specialist, we might say to the person sitting across from us something like, "If I can help you step back and get some space between you and the things that are bothering you, you might have a chance to come up with some new answers. Or at least feel a breath of fresh air pass through you! As it stands now your formed personality is a bit of a straightjacket, just as it is for everyone, and we want to release the grip of that straightjacket as best we can. So I want to sell you on this idea of 'executive awareness' and explain how you can cultivate it. Do you want to give this a try?"

This nonthreatening, nonjudgmental, potentially helpful tactic is the sort of tactic that a human experience specialist might employ to deal with the realities we've been discussing in this chapter: the conforming and conserving tendencies in our nature that prevent us from helping ourselves even though help is needed. Even if we must conceptualize the bar as low, that isn't to say that we can't also imagine ways of raising the bar with a given individual. It would remain to be seen whether our tactics would work, and it might be smart not to feel too sanguine as we begin. However, it might also be smart of us not to write the individual off and suppose that he is completely straightjacketed and unfree.

Free Will and Determinism

What we've been grappling with in this chapter are classic questions of free will and determinism. If we look at free will and determinism from the point of view of formal logic, it is easy to end up picturing man as not very free at all. Since everything is indeed "caused" in a technical sense, you can't do anything but what you do. What you end up doing has all these antecedent "causes" and reasons for existence. A certain causal chain, which is now in the past and can't be altered, produces the current effect. If you try to argue that your mind could somehow intervene now, maybe through "executive awareness," and make an important difference, the logical retort is that your thoughts are themselves "caused"; and so it looks as if you must remain trapped in some causal chain that can't be altered. This is the "strict," "strong," or "hard" version of determinism, and it can feel very compelling.

Here is how this strict view sounds with respect to our subject, mental health. Paul Edwards puts the matter beautifully in his chapter "Hard and Soft Determinism" (in *Determinism and Freedom in the Age of Modern Science*, edited by Sidney Hook):

"Let us suppose that both A and B are compulsive and suffer intensely from their neuroses. Let us assume that there is a therapy that could help them, which could materially change their character structure, but that it takes a great deal of energy and courage to undertake the treatment. Let us suppose that A has the necessary energy and courage while B lacks it. A undergoes the therapy and changes in the desired way. B just gets more and more compulsive and more and more miserable. Now, it is true that A helped form his own later character. But his starting point, his desire to change, his energy and courage, were already there. They may or may not have been the result of previous efforts on his part. But there must have been a first effort, and the effort at that time was the result of factors that were not of his making."

There is a sense in which this point of view can't be denied. But what's important to us is whether both of these people, the one who is free to be helped and the one who looks not to be free to be helped, can indeed be helped. That is, might some intervention now—something a human experience specialist could do, like introduce the idea of executive awareness and tactics for increasing it—become "just the right" new cause in even the unfree person's causal chain such that he gets mentally healthier? If this turned out to be possible, then we would have achieved the results we wanted, whether or not either of us—human experience specialist or sufferer—could be said to have been free to do otherwise. Looked at from this point of view, the question of free will becomes, if not quite a red herring, then at least a less momentous problem.

It doesn't matter if in some technical sense my decision to do the next right thing or the next healthy thing was "caused" or even "compelled" and that therefore I am somehow prevented from taking credit for it. Taking credit isn't the important thing. What's important is that I did the next right thing rather than an evil thing or the healthy thing rather than the unhealthy thing. If any of the following are one of the causes of my right action or mental health—wise early training, appropriate schooling, or the help of a human experience specialist— then all of those deserve support. If there are ways to help "cause" people to become mentally healthier, then we should want to support those efforts—even if that desire on our part to improve the mental health of others is in some strict sense itself "caused" and not freely arrived at.

There are reasons why, for example, you are putting that pill in your mouth. Your action is caused and maybe even compelled. But is there a chance for a different outcome? If, for instance, we educated you in a different way, presented you with some updated ideas about personal responsibility, self-efficacy, and value-based meaning-making, trained you in skepticism and taught you how to interrogate putative experts— if, that is, to the long and mysterious string of causes and effects that came together in that moment of you ingesting that chemical we added or subtracted this or that from your history, might you have a chance to stop the trajectory of that pill toward your mouth?

We should probably expect any given individual to be bound up in his personality and rather straightjacketed by it. We should probably expect him to be enough of a herd animal and insufficiently practiced in self-awareness to have only limited executive awareness available to him. We should probably expect only a marginal level of cooperation from him because of human defensiveness, because change is difficult, because we who claim to help may not be seen as trustworthy, and so on. Likewise, we must acknowledge the reality of causal chains in life, the extent to which we are more compelled than free to act, and admit that the sort of freedom that we would wish a person possessed—or that we wish we possessed—is likely a chimera.

At the same time, and despite these realities, there are things that we might try to help improve human mental health. We might intervene early on and provide children with the skills they need to, for example, increase their executive awareness. These interventions could become part of their causal chain and part of a happier outcome. This early intervening could happen at school, in the office of a human experience specialist who works with children, in an online setting that children access, and so on. Second, we could intervene today, so that our contemporary action became part of that individual's causal chain and made his today and tomorrow better. We could change tomorrow by doing something useful today, so that tomorrow it was "determined" that he felt much less sad or anxious.

Even a hard determinist would agree that these approaches do not violate the strict precepts of hard determinism. Even if everything is indeed determined, that doesn't mean that new outcomes can't also be determined. I've previously presented a picture of our human experience specialist leaning forward rather than leaning back in an attempt to help the person sitting across the table from her. One of the things a human experience specialist should endeavor to do by leaning forward is become a new link in the causal chain of the person sitting across the table from her. She wants to count and matter in that way. Wherever the bar was previously set for that individual, our specialist wants to raise it. With posture and attitude, our specialist says, "Let's make use of what you have available, as little or as much as that may be!" Even if there's a legitimate fear that only a little may happen, one can hope—and with good reason—that a great deal is actually possible.

12

The Human Experience
Specialist

The type of human experience specialist that I've mentioned, one that I'll describe here in more detail, will almost certainly find no place inside any medical model system. She will refuse to "diagnose and treat," and she will find herself excluded from the world of managed care, HMOs, insurance payments, insurance panels, professional trusts, "mental health parity" schemes, and the rest of the mental health establishment apparatus. To be excluded is not her desire but simply a fault of the system. Since she will be excluded, she will need to hang out her shingle as an independent practitioner and operate as life coaches for example do, as a needed, unregulated outside practitioner.

Can she actually do this, given that she is forthrightly dealing with "mental health issues"? Will society allow her to advertise her point of view and argue, for example, that "mental disorders" are made-up labels? Would she be wise to take such risks from a legal standpoint? Because she positions herself in opposition to what society currently holds as its standard of care—pseudo-medical treatment as provided by psychiatrists, psychologists, psychotherapists and other licensed mental health professionals—she could easily find herself in a vulnerable position, exposed to litigation and pressured to refer the person she is helping to someone with the power to prescribe a chemical fix.

These are big and perhaps unsolvable issues. But let's imagine for the sake of argument that these issues could be resolved—which, given how odd and diverse the world of helping already is, might not be an impossibility. Today a distressed person might visit a psychic or an astrologer. She might go to an acupuncturist or a homeopath. She might see her priest or her rabbi. She might chat with the woman behind the counter at the health food store. She might follow the advice of a blogger writing for some website. She might consult a self-help book or embark on a shamanic retreat. She might chat with her sister or her best friend. She might do dream work, scream work, past life cleansing, gestalt work . . . given this weird and eclectic array, is there no room for a human experience specialist? Perhaps there is.

Not only is there this eclectic mix out there—many psychotherapists already function as de facto human experience specialists. They fib as they fill out the necessary insurance forms and assert that the person across from them has this or that "mental disorder" and that in six or eight sessions "treatment" will be delivered. Having done their fibbing so as to get paid, they then go about their business of simply trying to help. They ask ordinary questions, make ordinary suggestions, share their observations, ask what hurts, react sympathetically, provide some human warmth, and recognize that life causes distress. They already function as human experience specialists, and maybe some of them will come out of the "mental disorder" closet and affirm that they are already doing this work.

Since the world of helping is already odd and diverse, it perhaps has room for our human experience specialist. She would step into this heterogeneous world and stake out new territory. She isn't a psychic, she doesn't have herbs to dispense, and she doesn't focus on marriage, binge eating, spirituality, or any other one thing. She does more coaching and teaching than a therapist, more investigative work and psychologically minded work than a coach. She says this at once outrageously large and also simple-to-say thing to the person sitting across from her: let's look at everything. Let's look at your personality, at how your mind works, at why you feel what you feel and do what you do, at what in your situation is really intolerable, at where you refuse to help yourself, at where you fib and exaggerate and cast blame, at everything. Let's get our hands dirty and investigate your life, every inch of it, if you agree to that.

For example, she might say, "Here's what we're after. I want you to get insight into your situation. I want you to articulate your life purpose choices and your values so that we know what you're after, how you want to represent yourself in the world, and what you think will make you feel proud of your efforts. I want us to hypothesize about what needs changing and what might reduce your distress and name concrete work that flows from those hypotheses. I want you to do that work, and I want us to monitor that work. If we have to change our minds about the direction we're taking, we'll change our minds. If our hypotheses don't hold water, we'll float new ones. I'll ask you to adopt a certain position: that life is worth living, that you are willing to don the mantle of meaning maker, and that you won't quit on life. Let's fashion some agreements and get our hands dirty. Okay?"

What if the person across from her says, "I am old. I am ugly. No one wants me, and I have no reason to live"? Our human experience specialist must have her responses at the ready. This is what she is trained for or what she has trained herself for. It isn't that she needs theories, pat answers, or homilies, and she would never dream of turning this lament into some sort of diagnosis. But she does need a way of responding, a way of using her heart, her experiences, her savvy, her intuitions, and her training. She can't sit mute, and she must go well beyond that easy out of the client-centered therapist, "And how does that make you feel?" She must respond—and she can respond effectively by keeping her eye on her posture: she must keep leaning forward. She may have no answers, but she has the radical power of engagement at her disposal.

She leans forward and engages. Psychotherapists lean back. Psychiatrists lean back. Our human experience specialist leans forward—so as to exhort, because she is interested, because the person across from her may be whispering, for all sorts of reasons. She leans forward even if the person across from her is leaning back or turning away. Whatever this human experience specialist's tactics—whether she focuses on teaching new habits, on teaching new skills, on pointing out patterns, on zeroing in on cognitions, etc.—whatever her tactics, her basic method is to lean forward and engage in dialogue. Because she honors that very little is known about how human beings operate, she doesn't worry herself about having the "expert" thing to say—she aims instead at being human.

This leaning forward does not mean that she becomes a patsy. She knows and remembers that the person across from her is a human being who may prove difficult and who may have his reasons for misleading her, denying her access, refusing to answer truthfully, and so on. At the extreme, a complete lack of cooperation on the part of the sufferer will prove a deal-breaker. If you are falling down drunk, if you are in what is called a "florid psychotic break," if you look present but refuse to listen, if you are in such a rage that you need to be restrained, if, in short, you won't cooperate or can't cooperate, that is a deal-breaker—at least temporarily. Our human experience specialist will not give up on you even if she can't work with you at this split second, but there is very little she can do for you at this split second.

This is one of society's grave dilemmas, a dilemma that is answered in ways that make us sad but that are completely understandable. If you are uncooperative in one sort of way—for example, if you are violent—you will get restrained, contained, incarcerated, or institutionalized. If you are uncooperative in another sort of way—for example, if you have secrets to keep or your way of being to protect—you will spend some disaffected time with a helper and likely continue on your present course. In either case, you are not helping, and your inability or unwillingness to help matters. Helping begins only if help is possible; and if help is not possible at this split second, a human experience specialist must know the best practices for dealing with that unfortunate reality.

As a human experience specialist, I must take into account that you may rage at me, play me, or tune me out, that you may arrive with a powerful agenda that has nothing to do with receiving help, that you may show up so lost in outer space or inner space that I do not even exist for you. With one person, this inability or unwillingness to cooperate will be obvious: he may be dead drunk or babbling. With another person, this inability or unwillingness to cooperate may be devilishly hard to discern: he may present a false agreeableness, he may point fingers and tell stories, he may deflect me, wear me down, or in some other way win what he sees as a contest to remain himself. This is all natural, predictable, and even ubiquitous.

As much as she wants to lead with compassion and empathy, a human experience specialist must not prove a patsy. Her job is to help, not to collude or get run over. She may have an abused person sitting across from her—or she may have the abuser. More difficult yet, she may have both in one-and-the-same person. Side-by-side with her desire to help is her understanding that "being human" has many sinister implications, including the real possibility that the person sitting across from her is much more likely to protect his darkness from exposure than lead with truthfulness and light. She must not forget what "being human" means—that is her area of expertise, after all!

Given that significant caveat, that the person across from her must be at least somewhat available, how will our human experience specialist operate? She will act as a guide of sorts, a teacher of sorts, a problem-solver of sorts, a sounding board of sorts, a coach of sorts, a confidante of sorts, a teammate of sorts. She will travel with the person suffering through difficult territory where neither knows for sure what they will find or even what exactly they are looking for. She will own a personal menu of tactics that allow her to offer support, frame issues, hold the person across from her accountable, and do the sorts of things that good helpers know to do. A willing person and a savvy helper enter into a certain sort of collaboration, use everyday language like "sadness," "anxiety," and "boredom," and work together to choose and even create language that serves the sufferer. To put it simply, our human experience specialist would do no particular thing except try to be of help.

The "No Labeling" Alternative

What she would not do is "diagnose" and "treat."

The human experience specialist as I envision her would engage in no labeling whatsoever. It is wrong to "diagnose" someone because he hates his job, finds his subjects in school boring, becomes paralyzed in the face of hard choices, or is made severely anxious by his lack of success. These and a million similar human experiences are not "symptoms of mental disorders" or markers of biological breakage. They really should not be "diagnosed" as if a medical event was occurring or as if an observer knew what was going on inside the person.

What then are the alternatives to "diagnosis" if the person is coming to us for help? Well, we could ask him what seems to be wrong and he might tell us. The simplicity of this transaction may seem "simplistic" or "superficial"—but why should it? Why should it seem simplistic or superficial to ask a person what he thinks is wrong, listen to his answers, and maybe make some suggestions based on what he tells us? If he fibs and doesn't tell us the whole truth or even much of the truth, well, so be it. We will have to deal with that possibility in wise and crafty ways or else maybe we will have to sometimes just throw up our hands. But he might tell the truth and we might have some good advice for him. Why is that an outrageous idea?

In this human-sized scenario, no "diagnosing" need go on. The straightforward alternative to "diagnosing" is not diagnosing and instead conducting a wise human interaction. Is this just not fancy enough to warrant payment and therefore a horror story to mental health professionals? If you are a mental health professional with objections to the current scheme, you may nevertheless still believe that there must be some alternative system that will allow you to give reasonable names to what human beings present. You may deeply believe that there are ways to create a taxonomy that at least allows us to be able to say the equivalent of "a dolphin and a human being are both mammals." Mustn't something along those lines be possible? Can't we do even that minimal thing? That really remains to be seen—but the answer may prove to be no.

When there are a million possible causes for a thing like a smile or a sigh, we can either lump everyone who smiles together and lump everyone who sighs together, creating categories of "people who smile" and "people who sigh," or we can create a million individual "categories" for each person who smiles and for each person who sighs. Neither activity makes sense or is worth the effort. Rather, we are obliged to take all those sighs and all those smiles as part of what the person across from us presents and abstain from creating illegitimate or unnecessary categories. To create categories just for our own sake, so that we feel that we are doing something that resembles science, is to act in bad faith.

Imagine that one person is sad because he has no life purpose, another person is sad because his best friend is doing better than he is, a third person is sad because his mate is cheating on him, a fourth person is sad because he can't get over his childhood abuse, a fifth person is sad because he hates his government's policies, a sixth person is sad because winter has lasted eight months, a seventh person is sad because he can't get his novel written, an eighth person is sad because she has become invisible to men, a ninth person is sad because he can't find the wherewithal to announce his sexual orientation, and so on.

The "naming" alternatives here are to create the category of "sad people" (which is what we currently do by turning "sad" into the "mental disorder of depression") or to make all of the following categories: "people who are sad because their novel isn't working," "people who are sad because their mate is cheating on them," and so on. Is either naming operation useful or sensible? Is it useful to lump all sad people together under one umbrella? Would it be sensible to create a million categories of sad people based on our guesses about what is making them sad? What would be the point to either naming operation?

Consider a second example. Imagine several unruly boys at a school. One is unruly because he is bored, a second is unruly because he is being picked on, a third is unruly because his parents fight all the time, a fourth is unruly to gain attention, a fifth is unruly because he's already a mean son-of-a-gun, a sixth is unruly because he finds math hard, and so on. To repeat, we can only do one of three things here with respect to naming. We can pin a single label on all these boys, using words like "defiant" or "oppositional" or "attention deficit disordered" and claiming that they all have the same "mental disorder." Or we can create a separate category for each "type of unruliness." Or we can admit that these boys really have nothing in common except one observable behavior. Either we create an empty category, endless categories, or no categories at all. Only the latter is honest.

Many professionals who oppose the current labeling system nevertheless believe that there must be some alternative labeling system that makes sense. Whether they want to retain the fancy word "diagnosis" or whether they are willing to give it up, they possess a belief that they can't shake that there must be some legitimate categories into which human beings fit. Aren't there really "hoarders" and "anorexics" and "alcoholics"? Aren't there really "pedophiles" and "cutters" and "schizophrenics"? Aren't these categories and many more like them reasonable, sensible, and useful categories? Isn't that just obvious?

No, it isn't—not at all. What if a "pedophile" is also an "alcoholic"? What if a "hoarder" is also a "schizophrenic"? What if someone is "anorexic," a "cutter," and also many other things, say "a fundamentalist," "an incest survivor," and a "classical musician." Which thing is she really? The idea that these categories are reasonable, sensible, and useful breaks down the second you look closely at them. It may be very hard to shake your belief that we need labels like "clinical depression," "alcoholism," "anorexia," and so on, yet shaking that belief is a necessary step if we are to effectively answer the question, "What should replace diagnosis?" The uncomfortable, even mindboggling answer is to not diagnose at all and to not create taxonomies of convenience.

Each person is his own story. No theory about him is true; no category into which you put him is a legitimate definition of him. This is the high ideal at the center of humanistic, existential, and person-centered therapy, that each person be considered a person, acknowledged as a person, and accepted as a person. What action plan flows from this way of thinking? I think a very simple one. The new slogan of our future mental health professional might be, "We try to offer people the help they want and the help they need without labeling them." This might become one of a human experience specialist's favorite exclamations.

That isn't to say that we wouldn't need strategies and tactics. We would indubitably need tactics to deal with all the tricky ways that human beings behave. We would need tactics to deal with the person who refuses to eat, who starts drinking at dawn, who can't get on a plane, who feels sad every day. We would need lots of tactics! To say that we listen and respond is not to say that we are sitting in some easy chair. But to say that we need tactics is not to say that we need taxonomies.

It adds nothing but an easy-to-use label to call the girl who refuses to eat "anorexic" or the man who starts drinking at dawn "alcoholic."

Of course, a human experience specialist would need to know these labels, since the world uses them, and it would be silly not to be able to find useful information because you didn't know the lingo. But that is a different matter from believing in the labels or countenancing them. The human experience specialist that I am picturing as the mental health helper of the future would know the lingo, would know about the special challenges with which "an anorexic" or "an alcoholic" is likely to be grappling, would know what seems to help best with those special challenges, and so on—she would not be opting for ignorance. But she wouldn't call the girl sitting across from her "an anorexic." She would call her by her name.

Helpers need tactics and not taxonomies. A human experience specialist is a tactician and not a diagnostician. When you sit across from a person and you want to help him, you don't need to know what to call him. You need to know what to do to help him. The place for diagnosing and treating is medicine—or car repair, for that matter. When it comes to the emotional and mental health of human beings, we must refrain from pinning labels on them just because we can. As far as that goes, we could label everyone. And that would help no one except those who profit from labeling.

Training the Human Experience Specialist

No training program currently exists to train human experience specialists. Therefore, let's dream one up. Here is one reasonable human experience specialist two-year master's level program, three classes a quarter and eighteen classes in all, with summers for interning. The interning would naturally be vital—imagine a human experience specialist program without experiences!

The main difference between a class presented in a psychology or counseling program and a class presented in a human experience specialist program would be that the class in the human experience specialist program would provide meta-analysis or critical analysis of the subject matter presented. If the DSM were presented, it would be to analyze it and not to swallow it whole. For anything that might be presented—psychological tests, personality theory, etc.—the twin questions asked would be "What do we really know about this?" and "What have we really learned from this?" Each class would be a lesson in skepticism and not piety.

Here are the eighteen classes:

1. Being Human—Who Are We?
2. Sources of Human Distress
3. Personality—What is it?
4. Listening and Speaking: The Art of Dialogue
5. Person as Individual and Person as Social Animal
6. What Helps?—Tactics and Strategies for Helpers
7. Meaning and Life Purpose—What Are They?
8. Qualities of a Helper—How to Be in Session
9. Psychological Formulation—What Do We Know About the Mind?
10. Context: Human Beings and Their Circumstances
11. Psychology Today—What Help is Being Offered?
12. Session Work—What Goes On in a Session?
13. Labels: Dealing With the Language of "Mental Disorders"
14. The Big Five: Sadness, Anxiety, Obsessions, Compulsions, and Addictions
15. Relationships: Intimate Relationships and Family Dynamics
16. Lifespan: Being Human over Time
17. Practice-Building for Human Experience Specialists
18. A Day in the Life: What a Human Experience Specialist Would Actually Do

Might a good program look different from the above? Of course it might. One program might take a special interest in life purpose and meaning and have a more existential flavor to it. Another program might take a special interest in social issues and matters of social justice. A third program might include classes about work with children and adolescents and have that as its special focus. A program might include a class on how to ask strategic questions, a class on the differences between short-term work and long-term work, or a class on ethical and legal responsibilities. None of this difference or variance would prove any sort of problem as long as a careful eye was kept on the central idea, that a person intending to do a new sort of work was being trained.

There might also be some sort of abbreviated training program for therapists and other mental health professionals who want to be released from the grip of the medical model and the constraints of doing "psychology" and who see value in adding a human experience specialty to their current way of working. Many in the profession are doing this work in a de facto way already, but they might love a little additional training and a new set of initials to put behind their name. Let us offer them that possibility and see if they are moved to come aboard!

Our human experience specialist is needed for all sorts of reasons. First among them is that virtually all current mental health practitioners—psychiatrists, clinical psychologists, family therapists, mental health counselors, etc.—are by virtue of their training and their very name obliged to focus on the mind of their clients and not on their clients' lives. A person is not a brain in a bottle and not a mind in a bottle. He has a life, a personality, and a world. He doesn't "catch" depression; he experiences sadness and suffers. Right now, he may ask for a pill because he thinks he is going to some sort of doctor. In the future, if he is provided with a new option, he may choose to visit a human experience specialist and bravely announce, "I need help with living."

13

Twelve Shifts for Professionals

In the previous chapter, I presented my case for a new helper, the human experience specialist. But that isn't to say that current professionals—clinical psychologists, family therapists, clinical social workers, psychiatrists, and psychotherapists of every description—would have no place in a better mental health system. Not at all! I would simply ask working professionals to rethink their model and their practices, shift from "mental disease thinking" to "problems in living thinking," and become more of a human experience specialist in practice.

This movement in the direction of human experience specialist involves a repudiation of the DSM. It involves a repudiation of the idea that "collections of symptoms" are entitled to be called by some made-up, medical-sounding label. It involves a repudiation of the idea that without some real investigating we know what, other than ordinary life, is causing a boy to squirm or a girl to be sad. It involves a repudiation of the idea that we can ever really know what is causing human reactions like anxiety and sadness and a simultaneous embracing of our ability to be of help even if we don't know. It especially involves a repudiation of the idea that some form of medicine is going on.

This movement away from prescription pads and made-up labels and toward honesty and clarity is comprised of the following shifts, efforts, and initiatives. In addition to the shifts I describe in this chapter, I provide a complete alternative procedure to diagnosing in chapter 17 and more keys to the mental health revolution of which you might become a part in chapter 19. Taken together, and if implemented, these will help you remove the "diagnosing and treating" shackles you are currently experiencing and lead you out of the dead end of a pseudo-medical, expert-centered practice.

The following twelve shifts will help you move in the direction of providing care that matches our updated understanding of what helps to reduce emotional suffering and mental distress. Some of these changes are relatively easy to accomplish (like double-checking to see what your license mandate actually is), some are not too troublesome (like routinely checking in on a client's life purpose choices and meaning needs), and some are rather more difficult (like completely letting go of "mental disease" thinking and changing your body language from expert leaning back to engaged leaning forward). But all of them are doable—only if, of course, you are interested in attempting them.

Twelve Shifts for Professionals

1. The first shift is not so much a shift as a check-in. What is the actual mandate and wording of your license? If you are licensed or certified, what is it that you are licensed or certified to do? You may discover that you have more freedom to act like a human experience specialist than you ever supposed. The licensing laws of each state are idio-syncratic—and often contradictory. In one paragraph your licensing law may announce that you are entitled to practice independently and in another paragraph it may state that if you encounter "mental illness" (which means what?) that you are obliged not only to refer to a medical doctor (psychiatrist?) but also obliged to enter into a "real" working collaboration with that medical doctor. These are the sorts of tortuous twists and turns encountered in all licensing language.

    Are you really obliged to "diagnose and treat mental disorders," are you somehow restricted to "handling psychological problems," or do you have latitude to frame your work as "dealing with the ordinary problems of living" and practice as more of a human experience spe-cialist? You may discover that you have much more freedom than you supposed and this new knowledge may help motivate you to make changes in how you practice your profession. Or you may discover that you are even more constrained than you had thought, which will prove an eye-opener and a splash of cold water in the face—and maybe an opportunity to become an activist in the service of change.

2. Shift in the direction of clarity and honesty. Get clear on what you are currently doing. What is actually going on between you and the people you see? Is the bulk of that nothing fancier than "chatting about life problems"? If it is, do you nevertheless rather automati-cally place such ordinary helpful conversations in the context of the "diagnosing and treating of mental disorders" for no other reason than that is what you have been taught to do or are accustomed to doing? What medical-looking activities actually go on in session? If the answer is none, think through how you might honor the good work you do while at the same time dropping the habit of "diagnosing and treating mental disorders."

    It is time to tease apart what you do because you think it is the right and appropriate thing to do, what you do because it is the customary and the accepted thing to do (even if it harmful, like handing someone an unwarranted label for life), what you do for your own ego, so that you feel like an expert and a professional, and what you do because it allows you to get paid, for example via insurance reimbursement. It is time to be honest and tease this all apart. This may prove more like an earthquake than a simple shift, but it is important and honorable work.

3. Make the shift in your own mind from "mental disease thinking" to "problems in living thinking." Rather than automatically ticking off squirming as a "symptom" of the "ADHD" or gloominess as a "symptom" of the "clinical depression," train yourself to ask yourself the question, "I wonder why little Johnny is squirming?" or "I wonder why Jane is gloomy?" Lead with "What's going on?" rather than with "What mental disorder can I detect?" Stop looking for mental disorders just because a shopping catalogue for mental disorders, the DSM, happens to exist and happens to have been foisted upon you.

    This may not prove a shift that you can accomplish easily or overnight, especially if your interactions with colleagues, HMOs, and even friends and family pull at you to retain a "disorder label" way of talking. What will you say if your cousin announces that his young son has some new sensitivity mental disorder and asks what you think about whether he should be accommodated or mainstreamed in school? It is going to prove very hard, verging on impossible, not to put on your professional face and collude in acting like this new sensitivity mental disorder exists and is a real thing. It is one thing to change your mind about mental disease thinking and as an abstract matter decide to repudiate it; it is a very different and more difficult task to make that change when you talk to people.

4. Make the shift from "I need to look like an expert" to "I need to be human." You entered this profession for many reasons, but among them was the desire to look like an expert, to be accorded the material and psychological perks that professionals receive, and to have your ego massaged by being called "doctor" or "counselor" or something similar. It is lovely to feel associated with medical doctors as a "doctor of the mind," and it is appropriate to be paid like a professional for the work that you do. But after all, it is rather like the work that anyone with human experience skills also does—it is what a sponsor in AA does, it is what a peer counselor in a high school does, it is what a wise aunt does, it is what anyone who understands life, who listens and who responds does.

    It isn't that you need to apologize for the fact that you aren't really doing medicine or announce that you aren't really a professional. Rather this shift is internal, away from acting like you know (which is the stance we want from our plumber, lawyer, or accountant) and toward the attitude of experimentalist, one who, like any scientist, has tools, tactics, tricks, and ideas but who, for example, doesn't really know what transpired before the big bang occurred until he really does know. A plumber fixes and a scientist asks questions. You can still be the professional you want to be, just shift away from plumber and toward scientist.

5. Shift your actual tactics, strategies, and practices. Think through what changes you intend to make in the way you interact with the people you see. Do you want to stop calling them "patients" or "clients"? Do you want to create a new sort of intake form that does a better job of inquiring into their current circumstances and their goals and aspirations? Do you want to ask different questions in session, respond in different ways, or propose more experiments? If you would like to become more of a human experience specialist, what would that look like in session?

That new, different look could take many concrete forms. You might begin to role-play and rehearse upcoming situations in session, for example, in order to help a shy person get ready for a job interview or to prepare a beleaguered mate to speak up for her rights. You might wonder aloud about what might be causing a sufferer's sadness, using a very ordinary vocabulary that includes words like disappointment, frustration, resentment, grievance, etc. You might present information, say about available community resources or stress management techniques, even if that feels more like social work, consulting, coaching, or teaching. In order to shift in the direction of human experience specialist, what might you add to or subtract from your current practices?

6. Shift toward a deep acceptance of the fact that you don't really know what's going on in and with the person sitting across from you and become much easier with not knowing. Admit out loud that you don't know, that the two of you are guessing, that your suggestions are more like experiments that may prove fruitful than like expert advice that comes with guarantees. At the same time remember that all this not knowing doesn't mean that you don't have ideas about what might help and tactics and strategies for helping.

We may not know what is causing a fire, but in the absence of counter-indications to do so, we think that throwing water on it makes sense. We may not know what is causing our shortness of breath, but in the absence of counter-indications to do so, we think that sitting down and resting makes sense. We act, but we also appraise: we throw water on the fire but register if the fire flares up; we catch our breath but we also register that our chest feels uncharacteristically tight and that we had better get right up, get to a phone, and dial 911. The same is true with respect to helping someone in distress. As we work with sufferers, we both act and appraise. We are able to act because we have a sense of what to do even if we don't know the chain of cause and effect confronting us.

7. Shift in the direction of paying much more attention to the role of socioeconomic conditions and other social and cultural realities in the lives of the sufferers you see. Better understand the power of

society to inflict emotional distress and exert control, as for instance when it labels a person for life with one or another mental disorder label. Recognize that "diagnosing and treating mental disorders" is a societal game. One year the DSM designates homosexuality a mental disorder; the next year it doesn't. That isn't medicine. It is the power structure making decisions about what is "normal" and what is "abnormal." Societal forces that control the purse strings and the paradigms positively or negatively affect your mental health—quite often negatively.

If you live in a society where every woman is a prospective witch just one wrong move away from being burned at the stake, every woman is emotionally and psychologically burdened by that prospect and that reality. If you live in a society where a key economic engine is slavery and you are the slave, you can count on despair. If you live in a society that believes that not to "medicate" a rambunctious child is tantamount to child endangerment, you and your child are on a collision course with the constabulary if you refuse to "medicate" him when he causes disturbances. Your society is your crown of thorns. Remember that as you work with people in distress—it may be society and not some "mental virus" that is harming them.

8.   Shift in the direction of advocating for a mental wellness movement that includes better conditions for everyone: less poverty, less hunger, less ignorance, less cruelty, more love—fewer of the bad things and more of the good things. Advocate for mental wellness and societal change in staff meetings, in blog posts, in conversations with your colleagues. Shift in the direction of advocacy. Advocate for the paradigm shift away from "diagnosing and treating mental disorders" and the pseudo-medical model and toward a "future of mental health" model where we all frankly admit how much we do not know and articulate how we can help a person in the absence of not really knowing.

Pick a particular hobbyhorse to lobby for. Yours might be teaching "life skills" in elementary school, teaching parenting skills to new immigrants (or to all parents), creating more communities of care, providing public service announcements that caution against the current ubiquitous chemical fix, or the "socialist" agenda of better conditions for everyone. If you fear that this general or specific advocacy will cost you your job or make life more difficult for you at work or lead to some other negative consequences, shift in the direction of bravery and heroism. Your mantra might be, "I demand more of myself and I demand more of the system."

9.   Shift in the direction of not flinching in the face of pushback to your advocacy and criticism of your new positions. One of the features of our species is that smart folks who do not want to tell the truth, perhaps because they have a financial interest in not telling the truth, can argue smartly against whatever a truth-teller is saying and embroil him in a time-consuming game where he feels obliged to answer each and every objection. When these carefully crafted distortions of

your position and loud objections start to come at you—about what a dangerous game you are playing by "preventing schizophrenics from getting the medication they need" or by "planting seeds of doubt about the helping professions"—try not to flinch.

Be prepared for this pushback. Your colleagues may well disagree with your position, feel the need to voice their disagreement, and even break with you now that you are in the enemy camp. Some of those breaks you may welcome, but others may cause you pain. A necessary shift to accompany your movement to your new position as naysayer and whistle blower is a shift in the direction of invulnerability to pushback. Simply offer your new proposals and argue for your vision of a different future. Say what you think is true, including fearlessly acknowledging all that isn't known and all that maybe never will be known. Rather than flinch in the face of objections or spend a lot of time arguing with opponents, stand straighter and fight harder.

10. Get clearer on the difference between a "difficult person" and a "mentally diseased person." It is absolutely the case that society can't allow certain behaviors. It doesn't matter what is causing the behavior: the behavior can't be tolerated. We refuse to tolerate drunk driving whether alcoholism is a disease, an addiction, a choice, a sin, or whatever. We refuse to tolerate the molestation of children whether a pedophile is a fetishist, is personality disordered, was himself abused, is bad to the bone, or whatever. We refuse to tolerate a dangerous "crazy" person waving a sword in public and shouting that he is a Knight Templar on a crusade, and we don't care if it is or isn't appropriate to label him a schizophrenic. He must be stopped. Society has the right and obligation to defend itself against its own difficult people.

But a provider ought not to presume that because a difficult person is difficult in one of these ways—drinks alcoholically, molests children, waves a sword while muttering, etc.—that it is appropriate to tack on a "mental disorder" label, as if by way of explanation. We have no idea what is going on inside these folks or what is causing their behavior. To add a label like "schizophrenia" onto what we are observing adds nothing and causes us to falsely believe that we know what is going on when in fact we don't. We can act as if we have done our investigative and explanatory work and wash our hands of the person by providing chemicals or prison bars. Our tactics for protecting ourselves against difficult and disturbing people shouldn't include making up names for them—as far as that goes, we might as well call them witches, demons, and ogres.

11. Shift in the direction of familiarizing yourself with the arguments against current practices, the experiences of sufferers and service users, and the many writings "in the movement." A suggested reading list is included at the end of this book that points you to scores of books worth knowing about. There are likewise countless blog sites, organizational sites, and individual sites filled with information,

including videos and documentaries. Among these valuable sites and organizations are Mad in America, the Clinical Division of the British Psychological Society, the Hearing Voices Network, and the Citizens Commission on Human Rights. There are many resources out there—get to know about them.

12. The number of shifts required to move from the expert/pseudo-medical model to the human experience specialist model—from the white coat model to the collaborative model—are many. I've described some of them in this chapter. However, the primary shift and the one that takes all other shifts into account is the basic shift in paradigm. The phrase "paradigm shift" is used rather frequently to provide added luster to a speaker's preferred way of thinking. Here, I think, it is justified.

When you stop believing that the laundry list of mental disorders that currently exists and the chemical dispensing that flows from that aberrant list are either right or proper and instead start believing that your job isn't to "diagnose and treat mental disorders" but to be there for another human being and help relieve him of his often severe human distress, that is nothing less than a radical paradigm shift in your way of thinking. It is the radical shift from looking for assorted leaks in the plumbing to acknowledging that life is difficult. That is the primary shift required of you.

There are more possible and useful shifts than just these twelve. You might shift in the direction of providing sufferers an actual document that spells out your beliefs and opinions about chemicals, diagnostic labels, and so on. You might have to shift your thinking so that you can picture a way of working where you lean forward more while at the same time maintaining good boundaries and keeping a safe distance. If you decide that it is time to transform yourself into a human experience specialist while still operating under your license, many shifts will be required of you. Create your own list of these necessary shifts—and start the shifting.

14

Institutions and Communities of Care

We need a new helper, the human experience specialist. But we also need new institutions and communities of care and new society-wide initiatives rooted in the idea that sufferers are not infected with some virus or dealing with faulty mental plumbing but rather are playing out their suffering in ways that make them difficult to deal with and that require an understanding of and tolerance for our shared human experience. We need ways of compassionately helping you even if you are very, very difficult.

If you talk a mile a minute in the throes of what is labeled as "mania," you are not easy to deal with. If you need your heroin and you also regularly want to kill yourself, you are not easy to deal with. If you are so wound up with bad feelings that you cut yourself or refuse to eat, you are not easy to deal with. If society could snap its fingers and say, "Please be nicer and then we will happily help you," it would probably snap its fingers. But there is no snapping possible because the causes of your suffering run deep and because your suffering is locked in, since that is what personality formation does. If you were easier, we would embrace you more, but you are not easy.

If we accept that difficult human beings facing grave difficulties are both things at once—both difficult and facing grave difficulties—we see why most institutions tasked with helping them turn into warehouses or prisons. It is easy to see why coercive techniques are employed to keep the caretakers safe and the sufferers contained. There is nothing surprising about the fact that if you are brought in kicking and screaming, you will not be offered a cup of tea, or if you are delivered after your tenth suicide attempt, you will not be permitted to keep your favorite belt.

Likewise, it is not surprising that your community is inclined to wish that you would just vanish. Who wants a heroin addict skulking around and committing robberies to support his habit? Who wants a crazy person wandering the streets and threatening children? Who wants a suicidal person stopping traffic as he decides if this is the right moment to jump off a bridge? What community is strong enough to care about its members with the kind of painstaking compassion required to help those unwilling to help themselves, especially when the members of that community are having their own hard time of it?

It seems like a romantic, utopian fantasy to somehow expect taxed, distracted, difficult and distressed human beings, whether they are members of a community or functionaries of an institution, to possess the compassion, wherewithal, interest, or skillset to deal with the most difficult and distressed among them, especially when the most difficult and distressed are also dangerous or seen as dangerous. The harshness of most institutions and the desire of most communities to expel troublemakers come down to something extremely simple: who really has the wherewithal to deal humanely with the most difficult, distressed, and dangerous among us?

Yet some people do possess that wherewithal and sometimes something different from mere coercion and warehousing does happens. Sometimes a deep, thoroughgoing desire to help people in distress translates into a way of helping that supports the dignity and rights of the individual, maintains a human and democratic relationship between helper and sufferer, and even produces remarkable results. Sometimes this is a one-to-one relationship, for example between a therapist and a client or between our future human experience specialists and the people they help. But there are also many examples of group efforts, efforts that roughly fall into the categories of community mental health services and therapeutic communities of care.

In the better future of mental health that we are envisioning, society would see these communities and institutions of care as worth supporting with substantial amounts of money so they could proliferate and become the new standard of care. A person suffering might turn to an individual like a human experience specialist for help, but might also join a therapeutic community for a period of time, receive help right at home from a helpful mobile task force, or check into an institution more interested in entering into dialogue with sufferers than drugging and locking them away.

There are many examples, both past and current, of these institutions and communities of care. One such example is the open dialogue approach to dealing with acute psychosis pioneered and practiced at Keropudas Hospital in western Lapland, Finland. In this approach, growing out of the work of Gregory Bateson, the British linguist and anthropologist, a team effort is made to understand the language and concerns of even the most seriously ill sufferer. Jaakko Seikkula and Mary Olson describe these methods in "The Open Dialogue Approach to Acute Psychosis: Its Poetics and Micropolitics":

"Dedicated to giving immediate help in a crisis, the basic format of the Open Dialogue is the treatment meeting, which occurs within twenty-four hours of the initial contact. It is organized by a mobile crisis team composed of outpatient and inpatient staff and takes place, if possible, at the family home. It brings together the person in acute distress with the team and all other important persons (i.e., relatives, friends, and other professionals) connected to the situation. The meeting takes place physically in an open forum as well, with everyone sitting in the same room, in a circle."

Later in the article the authors explain:

"As part of this approach, the question that a crisis poses, 'What shall we do?' is kept open until the collective dialogue itself produces a response or dissolves the need for action. Immediate advice, rapid actions, and traditional interventions make it less likely that safety and trust will be established, or that a genuine resolution to a psychotic crisis will occur. Hypotheses are particularly to be avoided, because they can be silencing, and interfere with the possibility of finding a natural way to defuse the crisis. The therapists therefore enter without a preliminary definition of the problem in the hope that the dialogue itself will bring forward new ideas and stories."

This approach, much more like "living poetry" than medicine, is rooted in many of the ideas we've been discussing: a thoroughgoing avoidance of "diagnosis"; an acceptance and acknowledgment of the humanity of the sufferer; an acceptance and acknowledgment of the fact that he is indeed difficult and that it is more likely that a team, where team members can relax for a moment while others take up the conversation, can deal with him better than can a lone helper; and the belief that an inquiry employing the language of the sufferer rather than professional jargon is absolutely necessary. The person in crisis is acknowledged, listened to, inquired of, and held safely by a group.

The Finnish model is one example of how better and more humane institutional care might be provided. The therapist Jed Diamond provides a second, quite different example:

"When I was five years old, my father tried to take his own life. Following his suicide attempt, my father was hospitalized at Camarillo State Mental Hospital. I still remember visiting him with my uncle. It seemed a horrible place with people shrieking madly or zonked out on drugs. My father spent seven years locked up there and I watched him deteriorate and become even more depressed and crazy over the years.

"I grew up and our lives moved on. The doctors told my mother that he was a chronic schizophrenic and would never leave the hospital. But my father escaped from Camarillo. He walked more than a hundred miles and took up residence in Santa Monica. An uncle unexpectedly ran into him years later and told me where he was living. I went to see him and was struck by two things. He was, as the song went, 'still crazy after all these years.' But he could also be kind and gentle and he put on puppet shows for the children in the neighborhood.

"He would seem normal for a while, but then he would become agitated and paranoid. His anger would escalate and he would become consumed by it. Eventually he would scream at me, tell me he never wanted to see me again, and threaten me until I would reluctantly leave. He refused to get help for his 'mental illness,' which I could understand, given his experiences in Camarillo. I saw him numerous times over the years, but our encounters always ended the same way. I eventually gave up having a father I could trust and moved on with my own life.

"Then one day I received an unexpected call from a social worker at Laguna Honda Hospital in San Francisco. They told me my father was hospitalized there and I could come and visit him if I wanted. They said he was in good shape now and had been there for three months. I was curious about where he was and how he had ended up there, but I was also reluctant to face the anger that I remembered from the past. I did visit and I found a man who had changed. His anger seemed to have melted away. He seemed happy for the first time in his life. 'This place has changed me,' he said. 'It's totally different from the concentration camp in Camarillo. These people really care about you.'

"It was only years later that I came to understand the healing that occurred in 'God's Hotel.' The physician Victoria Sweet spent more than twenty years at Laguna Honda Hospital. In her book *God's Hotel: A Doctor, A Hospital, and a Pilgrimage to the Heart of Medicine* she explained: 'San Francisco's Laguna Honda Hospital is the last almshouse in the country, a descendant of the Hôtel-Dieu (God's Hotel) that cared for the sick in the Middle Ages. Ballet dancers and rock musicians, professors and thieves—anyone who had fallen, or, often, leapt, onto hard times and needed extended medical care—ended up there.' My father was one of the fortunate 'creatively crazy' people whose wounds were healed at Laguna Honda.

"Dr. Sweet had the chance to practice a kind of 'slow medicine' that has almost vanished in our world. Alongside the modern view of the body as a machine to be fixed, her patients evoked an older notion, of the body as a garden to be tended. Fortunately, my father and thousands of others had a chance to be the beneficiaries of the slow medicine that heals body, mind, and soul. In a world of fast food and quick fixes, we need the medicine that Dr. Sweet was able to practice at Laguna Honda. Let the spirit of God's Hotel live on forever. We all deserve the chance to check in when we are in need."

We also have at least one example of something even rarer than the Finnish approach or the "slow medicine" of a Laguna Honda Hospital: an example of a whole community holding itself open to helping. Once in a while a living, breathing town decides to function as a welcoming therapeutic place. The place I have in mind is the Belgian city of Geel (Gheel), a community of thirty-five thousand that for centuries has provided wide-ranging foster family care for the mentally ill. Jackie Goldstein, a professor of psychology at Birmingham's Samford University and an expert on Geel and other therapeutic communities, explained:

"During the Middle Ages, the church was the primary source of 'treatment' for those besieged with various forms of what today we would call 'mental illness.' In 1249 the legendary Celtic princess St. Dymphna gained sainthood based on reported miracles and a belief that centuries earlier, in the region of Geel, Belgium, she chose martyrdom rather than succumbing to her father's mad incestuous demands. As a result, many sufferers sought treatment by making their way to Geel for intervention through the church and the auspices of St. Dymphna, the patron saint of the mentally ill.

"As those seeking treatment filled the church and the city, there developed a lack of housing for the visitors, whereupon church canons instructed townspeople to open their homes to the pilgrims. Thus was planted the seed of what would become an enduring system of foster family care for the mentally ill. Geel's legendary foster family care system continued to evolve over the centuries and even today, in the twenty-first century, functions as one part of a modern comprehensive system of mental health services, located in Geel and serving the entire region.

"In the United States, as we strive to implement mental health programs that promote community integration, it can be helpful to look for guidance and inspiration to the oldest continuous community mental health program in the Western world. For the individual with mental illness striving to live a meaningful life in the context of the recovery model of treatment, opportunities for community integration serve that model and are critical to its success. Successful recovery for individuals, in turn, allows them greater ability to function as members of their community.

"Geel's foster family care system is not necessarily a model that is appropriate for all communities or all clients. In fact, Geel currently offers other alternatives for care and treatment (another example of the community's flexibility). What is more noteworthy when looking at Geel is that the model allows for near total community integration in the absence of negative, myth-based stigmas around mental illness and real flexibility in the care of individuals with diverse symptoms. A community in this country might qualify as a 'recovered community' if, as in Geel, that community acknowledged the human needs of those with mental illness, provided social opportunities and meaningful work in the community, accepted those with mental illness as members of the community, and showed flexibility in its programs and approaches."

Geel is rather a special case. But many hybrid communities of care exist that are some combination of community and institution. Very often these are working farms; typically routine farm work is the cornerstone of the "treatment method" employed by the institution. These communities of care can't provide comprehensive or perfect solutions or handle every sort of sufferer. They typically restrict membership in the community and refuse admittance to, for example, sex offenders, arsonists, and violent individuals. They also often rely on what they see as the necessary, adjunctive help of "psychiatric medication." These limitations and caveats aside, these communities of care are very important for us to consider as prospective features of a new mental health system.

One such community of care is the Spring Lake Ranch Therapeutic Community in Cuttingsville, Vermont. Here is how they describe their services:

"Along with the opportunities for work and recreation, community is the backbone of the Spring Lake program. Everyone who comes to the Ranch has some essential strength that he or she can contribute to the community, and addressing challenging behavior in the here-and-now offers real-time reality confrontation in a caring milieu. In sharing life together, staff and residents alike open themselves to relationships that are reciprocal, rather than unilateral. Residents have a chance to gain greater responsibility and accountability in an environment where risks can be managed appropriately, and they become active participants in their own recovery. As residents progress and move toward greater independence, their community branches out to include other residents in our transitional living program and the greater Rutland community.

"The community aspect at the Ranch is most often visible at meals. Staff children and guests in the dining room add a home-like feel that is not often found in previous settings most residents have experienced. Holidays, birthdays and departures are celebrated with the entire community. The Ranch has many rich traditions associated with major Holidays, and we have created a few unique events including Yule Log Night, May Day, the annual all-Ranch Canoe Trip and our Harvest Festival. The Rutland program gathers its extended community together for holiday meals and special events.

"The core of day-to-day life at the Ranch is work. Many people who come to Spring Lake Ranch have lost the spirit and the stamina for work. When working together on a common task, it is much easier to make friends and focus on what one can do, rather than what one can't. On the work program, roles are fluid; residents and staff problem-solve on projects together, both giving and receiving direction. In time, self-esteem and confidence grow out of concrete accomplishment and individual contribution. Residents are asked to be reliable, on time, responsible and respectful—life and work skills that are expected in any job they may have in the future. Through work, residents become active participants in their lives once again in ways that are unpredictable, enjoyable, and transformative."

A second example is the Gould Farm Therapeutic Community in the Berkshires of Massachusetts. Here is how they describe themselves:

"In the year 1900, William J. Gould, a visionary and pioneer in social reform, conceived of a plan for emotional rehabilitation based on the principles of respectful discipline, wholesome work and unstinting kindness. Thirteen years later, 'Brother Will' and his wife, Agnes, purchased a farm in the Berkshire Hills, giving birth to the nation's oldest therapeutic community. Now, nearly a century later, Gould Farm's success continues to stem from the truth that a society is healthiest when its most vulnerable members are enabled to thrive. The Farm provides psychosocial rehabilitation in a nurturing and noninstitutional environment for adults (ages eighteen and over) coping with mental health conditions such as depression, bipolar and schizoaffective disorder and schizophrenia. Gould Farm is a diverse community of guests (our clients) and staff and their families.

"Gould Farm is the first residential therapeutic community in the nation dedicated to helping adults with mental illness move toward recovery, health and greater independence through community living, meaningful work and individual clinical care. Gould Farm offers a full continuum of care, with a Boston-area program for those ready for new challenges and structured transition. When guests arrive at Gould Farm they are generally assigned to work on the Forestry & Grounds Team. Team members get to know each other while tending to the woodlands, trails and grounds as well as indoor common living areas. Work includes lawn mowing, seasonal landscaping, splitting and delivering wood to the community's many houses, and maple tree tapping and syrup production. Instruction is given in maintaining and repairing equipment and tools for forestry and, as with all teams, coming to work on time, participating in team meetings and working with teammates are emphasized."

Compeer, Inc. provides a different sort of service. Here is their mission statement:

"Compeer Inc. develops, delivers and supports model programs that inspire and engage communities through the power of volunteer friends and mentors of our Compeer affiliate programs to improve the quality of life for adults, children, and families who strive for good mental health. Compeer Inc. provides supportive leadership to its community-based Compeer programs throughout the United States, Australia, and Canada. The objectives of Compeer Inc. are to support our affiliate programs through program expertise, branding, and marketing communication and to grow our current base of programs, by providing a cost effective solution to communities.

"Compeer Inc. envisions a day when all communities embrace individuals and their families living with mental health challenges; when prevention begins early with children and their families; when living, learning, working and volunteering in the community is given expression through the social inclusion of all individuals and supported by the power of friendship and hope. Through our time-tested model and evidence based practices of supportive friendship and mentoring, Compeer Inc. creates programs to meet the diverse needs of communities that want to improve and positively impact the lives of individuals and families living with mental health challenges."

Here are three of their success stories, as provided on their site: "Carol of Naples, Fla., credits Compeer with saving her life. Carol contemplated suicide many times before getting a Compeer friend. She writes, 'Compeer has helped me to stay out of the hospital and it has also helped me to maintain my stability. There were many times I was so discouraged that I would love to permanently end the pain—forever. I no longer want to curl up and cry. Compeer has made such a difference in my life; it is literally my support system and lifeline.'

"Jeff from Philadelphia made the transition from a mental-health consumer to a Compeer volunteer. 'I have been a consumer for more than thirty years, being diagnosed with schizophrenia a month before my high-school graduation. I know firsthand how it feels to be lonely and isolated, and I wanted to be able to help someone overcome these feelings. I believe having friends and doing things in the community builds confidence and motivation - and helps people cope with stress.'

"Loyd of Anchorage, Alaska explained: 'Isolation is the worst thing that can happen to the mentally ill. Isolation very often leads to death, while companionship leads to revival, the pure thrill of living. Volunteer companions in the Compeer program eagerly demonstrate that they care about their disabled friends, and slowly, but surely, return that glimmer of a grin back to their once distraught participants.'"

I have no personal knowledge of these institutions and communities of care and can't vouch for them. But I think it is fair to take them as suggestive of where we might want to go in some better future of mental health services provision. There is no reason why these and other apparent success stories shouldn't grip the imagination of some documentary filmmaker, and then, once his or her film is made, form the centerpiece of a video training program for institutional players and community leaders that acquaints them with more humane approaches to dealing with difficult people in difficulty. Wouldn't it be interesting to see the Finnish Open Dialogue Approach in action? Or take a "mental health tour" of Geel? Or have lunch at Gould Farm or Spring Lake Ranch? Such a documentary would amount to an easy first step in the direction of the creation of more communities of care.

A community of care looks to provide many benefits. First of all, it is a change in circumstances. If you got the chance to leave your unhappy circumstances—your family fights, your addiction triggers, your low-level, stressful job—and show up on a sunny day to a working farm and some friendly faces, wouldn't your distress likely get instantly reduced? Can't you, as a reader, feel yourself breathing a sigh of relief? Imagining the circumstances in which most people find themselves, isn't a community of care the equivalent of improved circumstances?

Second, there is the social aspect to these communities. We are individual creatures, but we are also social animals. It is true that we often do not want to be with other people, but we also crave community. Too much isolation tends to drag a person down emotionally. For someone in distress who likely is currently avoiding other people, isn't the opportunity to be around other human beings in this simple, non-judgmental way almost certainly a boon? It seems to me likely that it is.

Third, such communities of care provide a setting for individual growth and the possibility of a personality upgrade. Virtually all human beings have work to do to be more like the people they would actually like to be, more able to meet their own goals and live their intentions, and more able to take pride in their actions. If, in a community of care of this sort, you learn to show up on time, meet your responsibilities, negotiate tasks, and generally pull your weight, these new skills and habits, if they take, amount to the sort of personality upgrade that would help you become the person you would actually like to be.

Fourth, these communities of care look to offer warmth and support, key ingredients to successful therapy and what we all require. Warmth heals; support helps. Just as our human experience specialist is no patsy and keeps her wits about her in dealing with difficult people while at the same time leading with warmth and support, so too are these communities of care wise about setting limits and being careful while embracing and supporting the sufferers who come to live with them. You can be warm and careful at the same time; it is neither a contradiction nor an impossibility.

These communities of care look to provide these four benefits and many others as well. With billions of human beings suffering, the help and care they require can't be met by some limited number of human experience specialists or by some limited number of communities of care. Much more is needed, as I outline later on. A full-fledged revolution is needed. Those in a position to do so in society must institute huge changes if society-wide—and species-wide—distress relief is to happen. Be that as it may, we must not scorn small-sized steps like fostering a legion of human experience specialists and countless communities of care. They alone are not a complete answer, but they are worthy, valuable, and even essential in their own right.

15

The "Mental Disorders" of Childhood

Let's say that I am a school-age child and can't quite grasp a certain concept—say, multiplication—and to hide my embarrassment and distract everyone from my inability to multiply twelve times twelve, I pull the braids of the girl sitting in front of me. Is that a medical problem? Do I have a mental disorder? Or am I six months away from grasping a concept and in the meantime acting out?

For some reason (and we can name all the reasons) we have decided as a society that when I pull on Sally's braids, I have a medical problem called a mental disorder and that I should be obliged to take so-called medication to treat my so-called mental disorder. That is where we are today.

It is fascinating that whether or not my behavior actually changes by virtue of the strong chemicals I am forced to ingest, you, my parent or teacher, will feel relieved that I am "being helped" by taking that "medication." If asked, you will report that I am much improved. It doesn't matter if the chemicals I am given are inert and part of a placebo effect experiment, you will still report that I am much improved. My taking something has eased your concerns, and you now see me differently, as a good boy on meds. A lovely marriage of the placebo effect and the halo effect! I am much the better boy by virtue of taking something that is in fact nothing.

The child psychiatrist Scott Shannon is director of the Wholeness Center in Fort Collins, Colorado, a collaborative care and integrative medicine wellness center. He is also the author of two excellent books in the area of the mental health of children, one for professionals called *Mental Health for the Whole Child* and one for parents called *Parenting the Whole Child*. In the former he explains:

"One of the most interesting facets of ADHD is the placebo effect. Children with ADHD typically express little placebo effect as they hold little expectation about the intended response. It appears, however, that there is a placebo effect in medicated kids' parents. A meta-analysis confirms it. Parents and teachers express a placebo effect when children are given stimulants, because the adults hold a clear expectation for the medication's effects (Waschbusch, Pelham, Waxmonsky, & Johnston, 2009). Parents and teachers evaluate a child more positively if they believe that the child has been medicated. They also tend to attribute positive changes to the medication even when no medications have been given (Waschbusch et al., 2009). This finding diminishes the reliability of parent and teacher reports in evaluating kids for ADHD—the core of the diagnostic process."

We have come a long way over the millennia in our compassionate treatment of children. We no longer look at them as a workforce; we see them as having rights and deserving not to be abused; we believe that they have a right to be educated. Now, suddenly, in the course of just a handful of years, we have taken a huge step backward. As I write this, one in thirteen children are on so-called psychiatric medication. If you find yourself "in the system"—say in foster care—the number increases to one in four. And that number is increasing rapidly.

Because society looks to have swallowed hook, line, and sinker the pseudo-medical model that turns unwanted behaviors into mental illnesses just by saying so, we are on the brink of putting all of our children on powerful chemicals. Children are at risk; childhood itself is at risk. How did squirming in school or at church become a "symptom of a mental disorder" as opposed to an essential feature of childhood? How did sadness over the chaos around you, the constant yelling, or the break-up of your parents' marriage become a "symptom of a mental disorder"? How did disagreeing with your parents become a "symptom of a mental disorder"? How did any of that happen?

Let's say that you give birth to a child who comes into the world with a lot of energy. Should you maybe start medicating him at birth to make sure that you damp down all that energy so that he is fit for school and so that he can sit quietly in his chair when the drudgery of education begins? Say that you give birth to a child who comes into the world a little sensitive, a little sad, and a little anxious. Should you get her right on antidepressants and anti-anxiety medication and maybe some new anti-sensitivity medication so that she cries less, startles less, frets less, and is more like the child in the baby food ads, the one who is always so cute and smiling? Should we start all children on medication from birth?

Or should you maybe be a little reluctant to buy that your son's energy, your daughter's sensitivity, or your brood's acting-out antics are "mental disorders"? Should you maybe put your foot down and say no to the abolition of childhood?

Many of the "mental disorders of childhood" can be reduced to the following demand: kid, don't make so much trouble. Imagine that your child had the chance to talk to someone who actually wanted to listen, someone like the human experience specialist I've described previously or a good-hearted child psychotherapist who felt inclined to treat your child as a human being and not as a patient? Don't you think that your child's troubles might grow lighter if she had a chance to talk? Doesn't that seem like a first option and not as some mere collateral help to powerful chemicals?

When I was in second or third grade I pulled on the braids of the girl sitting in front of me. No doubt I was bored . . . and probably I liked her. She turned around and stabbed me in the hand with her pencil, causing a nice ruckus. I had to see the school nurse and the principal and, I think, was sent home for the day, either as punishment or maybe as a precaution. The faint imprint of that quintessential elementary school moment lives on at the base of my palm to this day.

Does that event sound like anything but childhood? If you are a parent, you have a new job in addition to all of your other pressing parental responsibilities: the job of standing up to the current hurricane of pressure to label your child with a medical-sounding "mental disorder of childhood." That is one of your most serious jobs, as that pressure is mounting.

As a society, as practitioners, and as parents, we really must reconsider the very idea of "mental disorders of childhood." We must make sure that we aren't punishing and ruining our children just because they aren't smiling, aren't behaving, have fallen a bit behind, are having a hard time of it, or find themselves marching to a different drummer.

Angry Johnny

In real medicine, you use symptoms to help you discern a cause, which then helps you pick a treatment. You take fever, fatigue, swelling, and so on as indicators of, say, a particular virus, and then you attempt to deal with the virus. If you can't discern the cause or if you can't decide between two or more causes, you run more tests and, while you are trying to identify the cause, you do things you know are likely to help relieve the symptoms.

In the meantime, as you seriously look for the cause, you work to reduce the pain or bring down the fever. You are reducing the pain and bringing down the fever while you continue to investigate what is actually causing the fever and the pain. You do not focus all of your efforts on reducing the pain or on bringing down the fever. You continue your investigations. You are trying to figure out what is going on. Your job isn't to merely treat symptoms.

One of our neighbors recently suffered from terrible stomach pains. For a long time, on the order of two months, no conclusive diagnosis could be reached among the four contenders vying as the cause of her affliction. Finally it was conclusively determined that it was cancer located in a certain stomach valve. Treatment began immediately. All along she was being given relief for her symptoms—relief for the pain, help with her inability to keep food down—while the cause was being determined. Treatment for the actual affliction could only commence once it was identified. That is how medicine works.

In the pseudo-medical specialty of "children's mental health" something very different goes on. There you take the report of a child's behavior—for example, that little Johnny pulled on the braids of the girl sitting in front of him—and for no reason that you can justify you call that a "symptom of a mental disorder." You collect several of these "symptoms of mental disorders"—often four is enough—and you attach a provided label to that "symptom picture."

The label might sound like "oppositional defiant disorder." Once that name is announced, chemicals are provided. Zero interest is shown in what is causing the behavior; zero interest is shown in whether the behavior reflects something biological going on, something psychological going on, or something situational going on. This is not medicine, no matter how many white coats are in evidence.

A child who loses his temper, argues with his parents, defies his parents' rules, and is spiteful and resentful is given, based on these four "symptoms," the pseudo-medical sounding label of "oppositional defiant disorder" and is put on chemicals to make him more obedient. This is not medicine. This is behavior control instituted to make the lives of adults easier. Why not ask little Johnny why he is angry and resentful? Is that such a preposterous approach? Why not step back and see if his family is in chaos? Why not look at his life and not just his "symptoms"? Why presume that a child arguing with his parents is caused by some impossible-to-find medical condition? Isn't it more likely—by a thousand-fold—that he is angry with them?

We don't know why little Johnny is acting the way he is acting. But we do not believe it is cause-less, and we do not really believe that it is the result of a medical condition. We must test for genuine organic problems like brain damage or neurological damage that can cause explosive rage, but in the absence of such biological challenges, we are obliged to presume that little Johnny has everyday human reasons for his anger. Once you rule out brain damage and other possible biological causes of rage, your next step should not be to posit a made-up, invisible medical condition but rather to treat little Johnny like a human being with everyday human reasons for his anger and resentment.

One fact alone should prove the absurdity of considering these behaviors a pseudo-medical "mental disorder." Imagine for a second that I said to you that my not being able to see any symptoms of your cancer was proof that you had cancer. Or imagine that I said to you that my not being able to see a break in your bone on an x-ray was proof that you had a broken bone. You would find those pretty odd assertions. What is fascinating is that mental health service providers are warned that they may not get to witness any of these "oppositional" behaviors because a child with this "disorder" is likely not to demonstrate any defiance except with his parents and teachers!

Unlike in real medicine, where the sore is visible both at home and in the examining room, with the behaviors associated with "oppositional defiant disorder" those behaviors are likely only observable when little Johnny is *actually angry*, namely at school and at home. It is absurd but true that an indicator that you have the mental disorder of "oppositional defiant disorder" is that you do not display any signs of it when you are talking to someone you don't happen to hate. Seriously, shouldn't the fact that little Johnny is only angry around his parents suggest that little Johnny is angry with his parents?

Picture what a provider is doing here. He does not personally see any signs of little Johnny's oppositional defiant disorder, and he takes not seeing them as further proof that little Johnny has an oppositional defiant disorder. He relies on reports of things that he has not observed for himself, things that are of course more logically signs of rebellion, protest, and anger than "symptoms of a mental disorder," and from those reports he "diagnoses" a pseudo-medical condition called a "mental disorder" and moves on to dispensing chemicals. He has not seen the "disorder," he has no tests for the "disorder," and he is basing his "diagnosis" in part on the fact that he has seen nothing of the "disorder"!

This is akin to the absurd claim made that proof of the presence of an attention deficit disorder is the fact that you do not display it when something interests you. Might it not be the case that you like to pay attention to things that interest you, like sports and videos games, and don't like to pay attention to things that don't interest you, like math class and your parents' dinner conversation? It is only through the looking glass that my interest in the things that interest me and that my failure to rage at someone who hasn't angered me are signs of some pseudo-medical "mental disorder."

There are many things we wish for little Johnny. We wish that he were having an easier time of it. We wish that he could stop his raging, for his own sake, since he is making everyone around him dislike him. We wish we knew what was causing his difficulties so that we could offer him help at the same level as his difficulties: if he is raging because school is too difficult for him, we would offer one sort of help; if he is raging because his parents are abusive alcoholics, we would offer another sort of help; if he is raging because he can't abide his parents' strict rules, we would offer another sort of help. We wish all of this for Johnny.

If a child has a medical condition, treat the medical condition. If a child is angry with his parents, do not call that a medical condition. Labeling an angry child with the pseudo-medical sounding "mental disorder" label of "oppositional defiant disorder" may serve adult needs for peace and order, just as prisons do. But it is not medicine and it is not right. Little Johnny is making it very difficult on the adults around him, who will naturally return the favor and make it very difficult on him. But that he is making life hard is not the same thing as being mentally ill.

We simply must stop saying that little Johnny is suffering from a mental disorder, that is, that he has a medical or pseudo-medical condition. It makes no sense on the face of it to believe that an angry child is angry because he has a disease. It makes much more sense to believe that he is angry because he is angry, just as you are angry when you are angry. Maybe little Johnny is a lot angrier than you are—but that he is angrier than you are doesn't turn his anger into a disease. As a society, we may not be equipped to deal with all of our sad, anxious, and angry children—but the answer to that shortcoming must not be to call them all diseased.

The Penalty for Squirming

The most common "mental disorder" to anoint a child with nowadays is "attention deficit hyperactivity disorder." This is the "diagnosis" you get if you squirm. The diagnosis naturally comes in different flavors—you can be "predominantly impulsive," "predominantly inattentive," and so on—and these different flavors exist so as to make sure that every possible feature of childhood is captured by one label or another. The unstated goal is clear: to turn childhood into a mental disorder.

Of course this "diagnosing" and subsequent "treatment" of children with powerful, addictive chemicals that resemble our "war on crime" street drugs is at once bizarre and, if the powerful could be taken to task, felonious. Yet the average parent seems incapable of saying no to the idea that common, understandable features of childhood should be transformed into mental disorders.

Would anyone put up with calling playing golf too many times a week if that negatively affected your ability to do your job a mental disorder called "golf addiction disorder"? Would you put up with telling the husband you hate and who disgusts you that you don't want to have sex with him a mental disorder called "sexual refusal disorder"? Would you put up with calling watching the same action movie ten times over a "violence attraction disorder"? Would you?

The funny thing is an awful lot of people would. Not only would people put up with such labels, they would likely embrace them and even crave them. It isn't that I like to play golf a lot—I have a golf addiction disorder. It isn't that I don't want to sleep with my husband—I have a sexual refusal disorder. It isn't that I'd rather watch *Terminator 3* followed by *Die Hard 2* than talk to my wife—I have a violence attraction disorder. I'm even a little afraid to name these "disorders" as a joke, as some readers will suddenly believe that these are disorders—just because I made up some names!

The mental health establishment has figured out that human beings in this culture at this point in human history will swallow such strings of words in a quick, deep, involuntary way, almost as if they have been waiting for them. Wish you had longer eyelashes? We have a chemical for your eyelash insufficiency disorder. Wish you had better taste in clothes? We have a chemical for your fashion blindness disorder. Wish you had a child who was zero trouble at all times? We have many disorders for you and many chemicals to take care of all that!

Imagine little Bobby who squirms at school, squirms at church, squirms at home, squirms in his good clothes, squirms when given chores, squirms when told to sit down and chat with his aunt Rose, squirms . . . a lot. What if you lived on a huge farm, it was always perpetual summer with no mandatory schooling requirements, and you didn't need to see little Bobby from morning until night? What would little Bobby be then? Would he be "ADHD"? Or would he be happy?

Wouldn't little Bobby zip in and out, make himself a sandwich, put a band-aide on his skinned knee, take a shower once a week or once a month, change his clothes after he fell in the pond, complain once a day about being bored, and be completely a boy? No one would be having any problems, neither you nor little Bobby. Where did the "ADHD" go? Where did the "mental disorder" go? Well, try to sit him down at the dinner table or in a pew at church and there it would appear. Imagine a disease only appearing at the dinner table, at school, or in church. What sort of disease is that?

The "problem" would, of course, return the second you tried to impose unnatural constraints on little Bobby's energy. Try to have him sit still during a sermon in church—now you have a problem. Try to have him sit still at the rule-burdened dinner table—"eat your peas first, sit up straight, stop fidgeting"—and you have a problem. Try to have him not climb on something that looks promising to climb. Then you would have a problem. Have you ever seen a child NOT climb on things that were there to be climbed on? Asserting your stubborn desire to climb on everything you encounter may well get you into hot water, but it should not get you a mental disorder label.

If you gave little Bobby the freedom he craves, would it surprise you if he popped in at three in the afternoon from his adventures to give you a hug out of gratitude for being allowed to be? Might he not even fail to fidget for significant amounts of time because he had spent his energy nicely being a boy? Would it really surprise you if he became the son you wanted him to be because you let him live?

Of course, I am painting a pretty and unrealistic picture. What if little Bobby's friends drank beer, used cocaine, and robbed your neighbors' homes? You would of course have to parent. You can't really let little Bobby run free—that picture of a huge farm and endless summer is a metaphor. In reality, you must parent. But there is a difference between parenting and letting little Bobby be labeled with a nonexistent "mental disorder."

Should a child learn to be orderly in school? Yes, for the sake of civil society. But that is a very different question than whether a child should receive a mental disorder diagnosis for not being orderly in school. There the answer is no. The issue of "being orderly in school" is not a medical one.

Doesn't a child have the right not only to a childhood but also to his or her individuality? Shouldn't a child have permission to say, "I don't want to be like you"? Shouldn't a child have permission to say, "I don't want to live like you"? Shouldn't a child have permission to say, "I don't want to think like you"? Shouldn't a child have permission to say, "I don't believe in you?" But of course, no child has such permission. That would be intolerable to adults. Parents would take that as criticism, as insubordination, as betrayal, and not as a right of childhood.

Such a child would be scolded, punished, belittled, and even hated. And, nowadays, almost certainly labeled and tranquilized. A child who fidgets is likely to get following messages. "You are such a burden to us because you fidget so much." "You are such a disappointment to us because you fidget so much." "You will never amount to anything in life if you keep fidgeting that much." "We can't love you if you fidget that much." In addition to those messages, which increase his unhappiness, he will nowadays get a label and a chemical.

Behaviors are not symptoms of a medical disorder unless they are symptoms of a medical disorder. Some honest person must fairly and appropriately distinguish between a behavior like restlessness that in virtually all children is not a symptom of a medical disorder, and signs and symptoms that are indicators of a medical disorder. That appropriate and fair appraisal is absent today. Someone with clout should shine a bright light on our current thirst for turning all squirming into mental disorders.

A Nine-Point Checklist for Parents

Rather than presume that your child has a medical condition or a pseudo-medical condition called a "mental disorder" when sad, anxious, or angry, presume something else instead. Presume that you do not know what is going on and that you need to ask some important questions of yourself, your child, the people in your circle, and, if they enter the picture, mental health service providers. Decide that you will think before you agree to allow your child to be labeled and "medicated."

Here are some questions to ask. This is not an exhaustive list. I hope that you'll dream up more questions yourself. Better to ask too many questions than too few!

1. Is there a problem?

   Let's say that your child is exhibiting some sort of problem. First of all, is it a problem? Is it a problem that your child waits two months longer to speak than did Jane across the street? Why is that a problem as opposed to a natural difference? Is it a problem that he enthusiastically signs up for violin lessons and then wants to stop them after two weeks? Why is that a problem as opposed to a change of heart? Is it a problem that he doesn't want to sit at the dinner table where you and your mate are always fighting? Why is that a problem as opposed to good common sense? You can call any of these a problem—a developmental delay, a lack of discipline, a refusal to obey—but where is the love, charity, or logic in that?

2. Who has the problem?

   If you belittle your child and he grows sad and withdrawn, your child certainly has a problem. But don't you as well? Isn't your habit of belittling him a genuine problem? If you are highly anxious and your child becomes highly anxious, your child certainly has a problem. But don't you have a problem as well? Isn't your anxious nature infectious? If you are rigid and dogmatic and your child rebels against your house rules, your child certainly has a problem. But don't you as well? Doesn't rigidity virtually demand rebellion? You can blame your child for his behaviors and take no responsibility for yours, but how righteous is that? The word "parent" doesn't make you right and the word "child" doesn't make him wrong.

3. What does your child say?

   Have you asked your child what's going on? Asking is very different from accusing or interrogating. Have you had a quiet, compassionate, heart-to-heart conversation with your child in which you express your worry, announce your love, listen to your child's concerns, and collaborate with her on creating some strategies and tactics that might help her deal with the problems she's experiencing? Are you in the habit of checking in with your child to understand what she is thinking and feeling?

4. What do other people say?

   Have you checked in with the people in your circle: your mate, your other children, your parents, and anyone else who knows your child well? What are their thoughts on what's going on? They may have nothing useful or productive to offer or they may have some very important insights into what's going on. Ask the people who know your child what they think.

5. Do you love your child?

   Human beings do not automatically love other human beings. Do you love your child? Do you soften in his presence and want to hug him or do you harden in his presence and want to scold him? Do you look at him with love or do you look at him to see if his fingernails are clean and if his homework is done? How reasonable is it for your child not to grow sad or angry if he feels that what he gets from you is not love but criticism and revulsion? This is one of those "looking in the mirror" questions that must be answered.

6. Are you quick to accept labels for yourself?

Do you regularly believe that you "have" something—clinical depression, say, or ADD? If you too easily agree that you have a "mental disorder" that requires "medication," it is reasonable to suppose that you'll find it easy to go along with the labeling of your child. If you say things to yourself like, "Oh, I have ADD and Bobby does too," "Depression runs in our family," or "We can't get Sally's anxiety meds right, but I've had the same problem myself," please ask yourself the question, "Isn't it time I really understood what a 'mental disorder' is and if I actually have any?"

7. Has my child had a full medical workup recently?

What if her school difficulties have to do with poor eyesight or poor hearing? What if her lethargy, her pain complaints, or her sleeplessness are symptoms of an actual medical condition? Make sure that you rule out genuine organic and biological causes for the "symptoms" that your child is displaying. This can prove a complicated, frustrating experience. The root causes of human behaviors are not so easily traced back to medical conditions even when such conditions exist. As complicated and frustrating as the experience may prove, a medical workup should be part of your plan.

8. What sort of help are you looking for?

You may well decide that you alone can't do enough to help your child reduce her experience of distress. But where should you turn for help? It amounts to a very different decision to take her to a child psychologist whose specialty is talk and who uses techniques like play therapy and to a psychiatrist whose specialty is "diagnosing mental disorders" and whose technical interventions are chemicals. There are many types of helpers, from school counselor to family therapist to residential treatment specialist to psychiatrist, who come at problems from different angles. Educate yourself as to what these different service providers are actually likely to provide.

9. What is the rationale for labeling my child with a mental disorder and prescribing chemicals?

If a mental health professional would like to give your child a mental health label, inquire as to his or her rationale for doing so. Ask questions like, "By 'mental disorder' do you mean 'medical issue'? If you do not mean 'medical issue,' why do you want to prescribe medicine to my child? If you do mean 'medical issue,' I would like you to prove it to me at least a little. And I would prefer that you do not offer up as proof that book, the DSM, which I am very aware is not a genuine manual but only a catalogue of labels and which I know does not offer up a whisper about causes or treatments."

Children are a vulnerable population. Their parents are their first line of protection. Taking your child's side sometimes means actively disputing conventional ideas about "what is right" and "what is best." The first step in defending your child's right to be herself and to have a childhood is educating yourself about the issues I've been discussing. You may agree with me or you may disagree with me; I put it in your hands to become the expert you need to be.

16

Understanding "Madness"

I've been arguing throughout this book (and how bizarre that it needs arguing) that human experiences affect us psychologically and produce important, life-altering effects. Living creates sadness and despair nowadays labeled and monetized as "clinical depression" and other "disorders of mood." Living creates worry and anxiety, today labeled and monetized as "generalized anxiety disorder," "obsessive-compulsive disorder," "attention deficit disorder," and so on.

Living creates other long-term and recurrent effects such as those labeled and monetized as "post-traumatic stress disorder" or "attention deficit disorder." Living creates addictive behaviors that are likewise apt to get a "disease" label. And living creates countless other consequences that do not represent pseudo-medical disorders or diseases but that are simply powerful human difficulties—often painful and usually unwanted.

So far I've left "madness" out of our discussion. I haven't chatted yet about those seemingly special and different afflictions known as "psychosis," "schizophrenia," "delusional mania," and other "serious mental illnesses" that affect perhaps 1 percent of all people—some new estimates suggest that 10 percent of the population sometimes hear voices—a percentage amounting to tens of millions of individuals worldwide.

Virtually everyone sees these afflictions as qualitatively different from difficulties like despair and anxiety. Most people suppose that if you are "mad," something in you has really, truly broken. It isn't that life has pressured you to hear voices, your genetics must be causing that, some neurotransmitter must be malfunctioning, something of that sort must be going on. It can't be that childhood or adult traumatic events acting on your sensitive personality led to such dramatic "breaks with reality." No, it seems clear that something has broken.

Yet it is rather more likely that exactly what we have been chatting about throughout this book, that trauma, stress, distress, and life itself produce profound difficulties and, in human terms, staggering consequences, is true for "madness" too. There is simply no good reason to suppose that "madness" is a disease, any more than there is good reason to suppose that despair or severe anxiety are diseases.

It is somehow clearer how losing a loved one or being faced with a horrific job might make one despair. But it is harder to see how repeated trauma in childhood might result in so-called "paranoid delusions" or "auditory hallucinations" in adulthood. Yet that this is harder to see is mostly a failure of our imagination and our empathic powers. We have somehow gotten it into our heads that difficult human experiences shouldn't bother us all that much. This is such a crazy idea that if you were a conspiracy theorist, it would cause you to wonder who has put what in our drinking water.

Could it be that we so lack empathy and imagination that we simply can't picture how addled we would get if we lived a life of daily trauma? I dare you to get raped daily as a child and not face a high likelihood that you will hear voices and end up with a "psychiatric diagnosis." When you get that label, you will be treated as if you had fallen prey to a "mental illness," as if some piece of biology had stopped working. Really? Was it really a neurotransmitter that got out of whack? Or was it all that rape that did it?

The clinical division of the British Psychological Society issued a November 2014 book-length report called *Understanding Psychosis* in which they argued along the same lines. They explained:

"We all deal with many stressful events in our lives—divorce, rejection, redundancy, bitter disappointments, bereavement and various kinds of failure. Even positive events—winning the lottery, for example—can be stressful. Some of us have more than most to deal with, in the shape of poverty, bullying, family problems, loneliness, abuse or trauma. Much evidence has now accumulated to suggest that like other mental health problems, psychosis can be a reaction to such stressful events and life circumstances, particularly abuse or other forms of trauma. A review found that between half and three-quarters of psychiatric inpatients had been either physically or sexually abused as children. Experiencing multiple childhood traumas appears to give approximately the same risk of developing psychosis as smoking does for developing lung cancer."

I have been arguing that human experiences produce more than mere "psychological consequences." They can rock a person, hijack a person, and disable a person. They can conspire to make a person "crazy" or, for that matter, conspire to make a person normal. As I mentioned in an earlier chapter, "normal" subjects in social psychological experiments are notoriously cruel. They will blithely administer electroshock to strangers for no other reason than that they are told to do so. This is "normal." "Normal" may be as problematic a state as "crazy." Are "normal" people who beat their children because their children are possessed by demons any less hijacked than someone who has conjured up voices to deal with palpable inner turmoil? Living produces profound psychological effects in everyone.

Life is an irritant, and our personality forms to deal with life's irritants. What we end up with are rocked, roiling, shadowy human beings, some of whom look "mad," the majority of whom give normal a bad name. It is much more likely that phenomena like hearing voices arise because of the way inner worlds get built under duress than because biology fails. Some anecdotal proofs of this contention are the ways in which the experience of war, the immigrant experience, sleep deprivation, and sensory deprivation can produce "psychotic" experiences. It doesn't look so terribly hard to become distressed enough to experience figments of imagination or to become disoriented enough not to know that you have created the voices you are hearing.

Consider the following small, trivial example, one with which we are all familiar. One afternoon you wake up groggy and forget for a moment that you are rising from your afternoon nap and think instead that you waking up from a night's sleep. Because you think you are waking up from a night's sleep, you know that the next thing you must do is make a pot of morning coffee. But making a pot of morning coffee strikes you as an odd thing to do, although you don't know why it is striking you as so odd. Something is quite wrong, but you can't quite put your finger on the problem. What surprises you is how large a sense of dread and dismay is growing in you as you wrestle with your confused, dazed state.

Of course what is going on is that part of you knows that it isn't morning and part of you hasn't quite figured that out yet. So, hesitantly, feeling rather weird about it, you take a step or two in the direction of the kitchen, so as to make that pot of coffee that you know that you really shouldn't be making. Finally the confusion lifts, and you realize that it is the afternoon, that you are not obliged to make a pot of coffee, and that everything makes sense again. You shake off your feelings of weirdness and return to your day, maybe still shaking your head a little at the oddness of the experience.

Certainly that wasn't such a troubling experience. Yet for those few seconds, you experienced something that is not a million miles from madness. You had a powerful inclination to make your morning pot of coffee as part of your inviolable morning routine and a just as powerful hesitation to do any such thing, producing, if only for a moment, a rather startling sense of disorientation.

Let's say, to pursue this example for a moment, that you reported your experience to a psychiatrist. You make an appointment and explain to him something along the following lines: "I knew that I was supposed to make a pot of coffee but some powerful compulsion or conviction in me said, 'Do not make that pot of coffee! That is the wrong thing to do!' I couldn't understand what was going on and it made me very nervous and anxious, if only for a few moments." What would happen to you if you made that report to a psychiatrist?

Well, probably that innocent report wouldn't get you a "schizophrenia" diagnosis. But don't bet on it. Your very appearance at a psychiatrist's office is a set-up for diagnosis. Don't be too fast to write off as absurd and ridiculous the possibility that you might receive a "schizophrenia" diagnosis in that situation. You may remember the famous Rosenhan experiment. David Rosenhan sent healthy confederates (a psychology graduate student, three psychologists, a pediatrician, a psychiatrist, a painter, and a "housewife") to a variety of psychiatric hospitals to see if they could get themselves admitted by reporting absolutely nothing except that they had heard a voice that seemed to be saying "empty," "hollow," or "thud."

These healthy confederates offered up no other "symptoms," concerns, or complaints. They otherwise painted a picture of a completely normal, healthy life. What happened? All were admitted, all received a schizophrenia diagnosis, none were immediately released even after they explained that they no longer heard the voice in question, and all were discharged with a "schizophrenia in remission" diagnosis. They had all become "schizophrenics" for life. When we realize how many people have the not-so-unusual experience of hearing voices— the authors of the *Understanding Psychosis* report assert that "up to 10 percent of the general population hear voices at some point in their life"—and how just hearing voices can get you a lifelong psychiatric label, we see once again why we are obliged to fight the current system.

So what is actually going on with "madness"? Of course we are not talking about mere disorientation of the sort we might experience upon waking up from a nap. We are talking about often severe and disabling difficulties that can leave a person isolated, frightened, unable to work, unable to function, at odds with friends, loved ones, and society. They can be agitated, raw, despairing, and suicidal. Many people seem to experience their voices as benign, and for them their voices may have arisen from a different place and for different reasons. Some individuals would argue that they are not suffering but are instead having a spiritual experience, an experience of growth and healing, or some other beneficial experience. But let's keep our focus for the moment on those folks who "look mad" and would say that they are having a hard time of it. What's going on with them?

No one knows. *No one knows.* The following, however, is one version, vision, model, or hypothesis of what may be going on for some people who start to hear voices that they believe are actual other voices. We'll leave for another discussion whether folks who hear voices "sort of know" that these aren't really the voices of others—many retrospective reports of voice-hearers indicate that they possessed a rather clear understanding that these were just and exactly their own thoughts even as they felt compelled to believe them to be the voices of others.

These folks seemed to have a pressing need to portray their voices to the world as the voices of others so as to give the voices more credibility—or to give their pain and distress more credibility. Whether this is a general rule or whether these are special cases is a question for another conversation. But we should keep in mind that we do not know even this much; that is, we do not know what a person who claims to be hearing voices really thinks about those voices.

The following is one vision of what may be going on. It posits a person with a certain habit, affinity, personality style, bit of original personality, cognitive style—call it what you will—that I am dubbing the habit of in-dwelling. As a child already, this person not only loves to spend time in his own head, he really isn't very comfortable anywhere else. Let's call our in-dweller John. John has a vivid imagination, dreams up fantasies and stories for himself, draws cartoons of other worlds, and even as a child has precious little use for what he disparagingly calls the real world. In that real world mostly hellish things go on; and those things that aren't hellish strike him as deathly boring. Because he experiences the real world as either hellish or boring, he avoids it as best he can.

John's mother overpraises him and tells him that he is her little genius and destined to change the world. His father belittles him and verbally attacks him. That his mother praises him but does not protect him from his father's verbal abuse is maddening to him: why not protect him a little more and praise him a little less? Because this makes no sense to him—wouldn't you protect the person destined to change the world, if you meant it?—he both despises her and refuses to believe her message, that he is super-worthy. Oddly enough, all of her praise produces a so-to-speak inferiority complex.

At the same time, he does feel special since he knows that the stories he tells himself are indeed good and lively, that his cartoons are lively too, and that he does have some spark or gift different from his boring little peers. He in-dwells more, relentlessly hides out, and pays less and less attention to the doings at school or in his family. His sense of agitation, frustration, and sleeplessness mount, and in the course of events, he builds up an impressive lack of motivation to do his schoolwork because his schoolwork bores him silly. He starts to almost fail at school, pulling off barely passing grades just so as not to create too much of a storm at home.

He also starts to build up an impressive lack of coping skills, since he hides out so much and interacts so little with his peers, and an impressive lack of decisiveness, since he can turn any issue over in his head a million ways and see everything from too many angles. His grandiosity increases as he fills notebooks up with what he believes to be brilliant cartoons and aphorisms, and his sense of inferiority increases as he is snickered at more by his peers and belittled more by his father. He becomes a kind of god-bug: superhuman when he draws cartoons, easy to squash in the real world.

John is a sensitive boy who is regularly belittled, pressed to succeed, told that he is worthless, told that he is special, who spends great stretches of time in his room because the world feels dangerous, because he is awkward around his peers, and because he is in the habit of staring at his ceiling and thinking obsessively about this and that. This pattern of in dwelling becomes habitual, and it has the pleasant feeling of habit while feeling completely unpleasant. This is because a part of him knows exactly to what extent he is hiding out and not living. He has no friends. He has no dates. He shares in nothing that everyone else at school seems to share in. His in dwelling is habitual, comforting, and pleasant up to a point. At the same time he feels ruined.

Has he already started to hear voices? Maybe. But if he hasn't, we surely see the handwriting on the wall and fully expect John to be already sad (i.e., suffering from "childhood depression"), anxious (i.e., afflicted with an "obsessive-compulsive disorder"), and odd. Maybe he isn't hearing voices yet, but isn't he a likely candidate? And when will the voices arrive? Probably when he experiences life as even more stressful than it feels currently. Let's add significantly more stress to John's life and imagine him finishing high school by the skin of his teeth and then entering into one of two situations known to produce their share of "psychosis": a war and the first year of college.

John is not likely to enlist in wartime, but if he is drafted, doesn't he seem a likely candidate for "battle fatigue"? Looking back at the World War II experience, Samuel Paster wrote in the July, 1948, issue of the *Journal of Nervous and Mental Disease*: "The number of patients admitted to army hospitals with neuropsychiatric disorders during the period January 1, 1942 through June 30, 1945 reached approximately one million. Approximately 7 percent of these patients were psychotic. Most of the patients who developed psychotic reactions during the last war became incapacitated prior to shipment overseas, often during the period of basic training. Many men, however, distinguished themselves in the service as well as on the field prior to the onset of their illness."

Can't we picture John in boot camp, thrust among "rough youth," yelled at and bullied by drill sergeants, and obsessing about his possible horrible injury or death, "breaking" under that stress, and starting to hear voices? But of course, it is much more likely that he will go off to college than find himself in a war, and it is that stressful first year of college, filled with the dislocation of leaving home, a cramped space filled with roommates, the simultaneous intensity and meaninglessness of his classes, and the odd demand that he "pick a major" when he has no idea what his life is meant to be about, that produces so many "psychotic breaks" in college freshmen and sophomores. Can't we feel how John might "cope" with the college experience by conjuring up voices?

In any event, when and if John experiences his "psychotic break," he is likely to end up in a psychiatrist's office. We must leave John there, on his first (but not last) visit to a psychiatrist. We know full well what will happen. Little or nothing of John's actual experience will get aired in the typically brief amount of time, nowadays on the order of fifteen minutes, that John will spend with this psychiatrist. John will receive a diagnosis of "schizophrenia" or something similar, chemicals called medication, and, if the psychiatrist suspects that John is a "threat to himself or to others," a commitment order. John will acquire a lifetime label and, as likely as not against his will, be forced into the system.

Is the picture I'm painting of John's slide indeed what happens? Is this the process or perhaps one version of the process? Can we say for sure that circumstances of this sort combined with a temperament of this sort would produce any consequences in particular: sadness, anxiety, hearing voices, etc.? We do not know. But it is surely a reasonable and intuitively sensible possibility, isn't it? And it is certainly illegitimate, arrogant, and cruel to announce that John has a medical condition called "mental illness" just because that is the current paradigm. We must stop labeling people with medical conditions when the causes of their distress have no connection to any known medical problem.

We must stop saying, "You have schizophrenia," when what we mean is, "We don't know."

We do not know enough about what is going on with John. What we do know for certain is that adding the medical-sounding label of schizophrenia to a situation like John's adds nothing and comes with a stupendous cost. What costs? As the authors of the *Understanding Psychosis* report put it, "Receiving a diagnosis can also have negative psychological effects on the person, for example leading to feelings of hopelessness and decreased confidence. It can give the message that people can do little to overcome their problems except to 'keep taking the tablets'. It can divert attention from the possible meaning or positive aspects that the experiences might have for the person. It can also deflect attention away from underlying social and emotional problems that could otherwise be addressed in a restorative way, for example the aftermath of adversities like poverty, discrimination, childhood abuse or assault. Importantly, the way that diagnoses *appear* to summarize the nature and causes of someone's experience can prevent workers from asking about, and helping the person to deal with the events and emotions that may in reality underlie the problems."

The main problem we have with accepting the possibility that you can hear voices without having an organic or biological problem is that we can't conceive of it or imagine it. But that is our problem. Consider what may be completely analogous phenomena, "psychogenic pain" and "hysterical blindness." In the first case, a person experiences genuine pain, pain as real as pain can be, without any underlying organic or biological problem. In the second case, a person really can't see—really can't see—even though there is no underlying organic or biological problem. For instance, a significant number of pilots in wartime who could no longer tolerate the stress of imminent death became blind in this way.

In the cases of psychogenic pain and hysterical blindness, we intuit how a psychological situation is able to produce an odd physical symptom that is usually caused by biological, organic, or anatomical reasons. We get it. If we just let our imagination leap to what may be an exact analogy, we might grow easier with the idea that a phenomenon like hearing voices need have no biological or organic cause either. It may arise just as psychogenic pain or hysterical blindness arises in a human being who is stressed beyond his or her limits.

It makes perfect sense that a person might believe that the problem is organic or biological, just as a person experiencing psychogenic pain or hysterical blindness may not be able to be convinced that his affliction isn't "real" and that it only "exists in his head." So we must take this natural defensiveness into account with a person who is in pain in this way, who is blind in this way, or who hears voices in this way and who asserts—who insists—that he has a disease or a biological or organic problem. It should be easy enough to imagine how hearing voices could arise in this fashion and why the person hearing voices might insist that the voices are real, just as a wartime pilot insists that his blindness is real.

What I am talking about must, of course, be distinguished from the sorts of auditory and visual hallucinations that arise for biological reasons. A psychological slant must not be put on essentially biological phenomena. But by the same token, a biological slant should not be put on essentially psychological phenomena. Likewise, I am not trying to ascribe blame nor do I mean to let "mad" people off the hook. I've already spent a chapter explaining that human beings are difficult. They are difficult whether they are "normal," "mad," or anything in between. These are separate questions.

We tend to want to hold "mad" people less responsible than their "normal" counterparts, but it remains an open question as to what extent they can or can't reasonably be held responsible. If it is the case that sometimes a "mad" person massages his madness so as not to have to deal with his problems—his lack of employment and his resistance to employment, the nonsense of the real world, and so on—and if in fact his break with reality is less a complete break and more a fracture through which reality can be seen through the cracks, then ought we demand that he take some responsibility for his state and his difficulties? These are important but separate questions.

All of your life you have heard that there is something called the "mental illness" of "schizophrenia" and, without giving it much or any thought, you have likely presumed that this means that a "crazy person" must have some unfortunate biological malfunction like a genetic indictment, a brain anomaly, a neurotransmitter problem, and so on. This view is being hotly disputed and may prove completely false. It may well turn out that hearing voices, for example, which is one of the hallmarks of "psychosis," is simply one predictable result of a childhood that is experienced as traumatic by a person who possesses the habit of in-dwelling. Because this possibility may be true, we ought to provide help that really helps this person—which, to begin with, involves just listening.

As the authors of the *Understanding Psychosis* report conclude, "Hearing voices and feeling paranoid are common experiences which can often be a reaction to trauma, abuse or deprivation. Calling them symptoms of mental illness, psychosis or schizophrenia is only one way of thinking about them . . . The causes of a particular individual's difficulties are always complex. Our knowledge of what might have contributed, and what might help, is always tentative. Professionals need to respect and work with people's own ideas about what has contributed to their problems . . . Professionals should not promote any one view, or suggest that any one form of help such as medication or psychological therapy is useful for everyone. Instead we need to support people in whatever way they personally find most helpful."

We do not know what "madness" is or what it represents, but we add nothing when we call it "psychosis" or "schizophrenia" and act like we do know. Rather than adding, we subtract. We subtract energy from all sorts of new research that might help us understand the relationship between human experience and phenomena like hearing voices. We subtract good will and incline ourselves toward a model of compulsion and coercion. We subtract empathy and promote a vision of "us" and "them": us as normal and them as crazy. All this subtracting costs lives. Let us try to be of more help, even from the unfortunate place of not knowing enough, and stop labeling when we ought to be caring.

17

Alternatives to Diagnosis

Those of us who do not believe in the pseudo-medical model of mental health service provision want all of the following to happen:

1. We want to help deconstruct and rid society of the "mental illness" model and "mental illness thinking."
2. We want specifically to dispute the DSM, its paradigm, and the medicalization of society that flows from that paradigm (including wanton chemical dispensing).
3. We want to provide folks in distress with a different vision from the pseudo-medical one and a different road back from suffering than "just meds." We want this to include "talk," but we want this to be talk about everything that matters to the person, including talk about things that are not strictly "psychological."
4. Ultimately we want to produce a replacement paradigm to the DSM/ pseudo-medical model that is intellectually more honest, genuinely more helpful, practical enough that it can be "communicated easily" (whether for insurance purposes or just so that two human beings can have a conversation), and that will find favor with practitioners.
5. We want that paradigm to include "more of life" than most current models do (whether that current model is a pseudo-medical sort of model or a psychological sort of model): we want socioeconomic realities included, we want life circumstances included, we want existential realities included, and so on. We want to create a paradigm that "includes psychology" but that also moves "beyond psychology" to include everything pertinent to an understanding of human distress and human helping.
6. We want to make it clear that it makes no sense to "buy" any particular psychological theory, model, or paradigm as the be-all and end-all, whether that model is a CBT one, a Jungian one, and so on; and that while we are ecumenical enough to suppose that any particular psychological theory, model, or paradigm might have interesting things to say and useful practices to aid a service provider, we want to make it clear that there is no existing paradigm that can be considered a winner. Each, because of the nature of the task at hand—fully understanding human beings—only deals with the trunk or the tail of the elephant (or only deals with one version of the elephant).

171

Introducing a "Life Formulation Model"

Taking all of the above into consideration, I think that the following makes sense as an alternative to the current models and paradigms. I am calling it a "life formulation model." It nicely disputes the current DSM paradigm and also frees us from the tyranny of acting as if we are talking only about "psychology" when we talk about mental health, when in fact we are talking about all of life.

In this life formulation model, a practitioner would describe her relationship with the person she is seeing in six ways: 1) the person's expressed concerns; 2) the person's circumstances of note; 3) the person's behavioral and emotional considerations; 4) the person's challenges as inferred by the provider; 5) the provider's concerns; and 6) the provider's recommendations. There would be no DSM or pseudo-medical language used in this model, no new diagnostic language introduced, and everything would be described in "plain English" (or plain French or plain German).

How might this work? Let's consider a fifteen-year-old girl named Jane who is "brought in" to a service provider by her parents. They believe that Jane is "depressed." They are also worried about her drinking, her insomnia, her school difficulties, her thinness, and the fact that she is cutting herself.

First the service provider would check in with Jane about Jane's expressed concerns. These might turn out to be that Mary likes Elizabeth better than she likes Jane; that the clique that includes Mary and Elizabeth will not let Jane in; that Billy prefers Elizabeth to Jane; that Mrs. Williams in English may well be giving Jane a C, ruining Jane's chances of getting into the college she is dreaming of attending; and that her parents are driving her crazy by always scrutinizing her and criticizing her.

There is absolutely no reason why these concerns can't also come with some sort of number, if that were deemed useful: it would not be hard to create a huge list of concerns and attach a number to each one, if that was wanted. So let's say that in addition to the words describing Jane's concerns, there were also numbers: let's say 1104, 1931, 2242, 4482 and 5561. It would be child's play to list those five numbers in a "summary report," if a service provider needed to do such a thing. This would look like: Expressed Concerns (1104, 1931, 2242, 4482, 5561). (I think there is a better way to do this summarizing, which I will describe later.)

Next would come an acknowledgment and understanding of Jane's circumstances as gleaned from Jane and maybe from the reports of others. This might sound like:

Circumstances of Note:

- In Jane's family, a college education and a professional career are required
- In Jane's family, it is not permitted to date someone from a different cultural or religious background
- Jane is not permitted to lock her door or any door, including the bathroom door
- Jane surprised herself by doing much more poorly in freshman year that she had expected
- Jane's older sisters were the stars of her high school

Are these all the circumstances one might include? Of course they aren't. Are these the most pertinent circumstances to include? Who knows? But each is suggestive and each helps a service provider understand Jane's reality. They may not be exactly the correct circumstances to note or a sufficient number of circumstances to note, but they are important and they matter.

Next would come behavioral and emotional considerations. In Jane's case, this might look like the following:

- Jane is cutting herself (confirmed by Jane)
- Jane is drinking excessively (disputed by Jane)
- Jane is quite sad (confirmed by Jane)
- Jane is starving herself (disputed by Jane)
- Jane is sleeping very little (confirmed by Jane)

Next would come inferred challenges, that is, the provider's ideas about what is going on. This might sound like the following:

- Predictable challenges of adolescent girls in Jane's cultural and socio-economic situation
- Special challenges of living in a strict, punitive family
- Emotional challenges of intense sadness and constant worry
- Cognitive challenges of self-denigrating and punitive self-talk
- Behavioral challenges of cutting, drinking, starvation and sleeplessness

These inferred challenges would be described in the service provider's preferred language: the language of psychological formulation, the language of narrative psychology, the language of CBT, the language of Jung, the language of Freud or contemporary psychoanalysis, the language of existential psychotherapy, in "ordinary" or "everyday" language, and so on.

You could use any language, indicating where the language came from: that is, in addition to a long list of everyday inferences (like "the predictable challenges of adolescence") there might be also long lists of Jungian inferences, existential inferences, etc. If a code was needed, coded items might appear as J462 for "Jungian mid-life crisis" or F993 for "Freudian arrested development in the anal stage" and so on. Naturally (and hopefully) these taxonomical niceties would not be needed or wanted. But if they were, they could be accommodated.

Next would come the provider's concerns. These would be expressed in ordinary language in the following sort of way:

- Concerned that Jane has no one to talk to, given that she's on the outs with her successful siblings and that she has no confidante in either of her parents
- Wondering if Jane was born a little sad and, if so, if sadness will constitute a lifelong challenge for her
- Some suspicions of childhood sexual abuse given Jane's particular presentation
- Want to really focus on the sleeplessness and its causes, as sleeplessness can drive "mania" and "psychosis"
- Must tackle the cutting, the drinking, and the self-starvation

Next would come the provider's recommendations. This might sound like:

- Cognitive work around self-esteem
- Depth work around possible trauma
- Behavioral work around eating, cutting, and drinking
- Behavioral work around sleeping
- Family work around expectations

Personally I would want a seventh category that communicates the sufferer's life purposes, dreams, goals, aspirations, and other existential and motivational factors. These could be reported in ordinary language and might sound like the following:

- Jane remembers her camp counseling experiences as particularly meaningful
- Jane considers that one of her life purposes is to marry and raise a family although she believes that she would be a "bad parent"

- Jane would like to leave her small town and live in London or Paris
- Jane sees herself as both "secular" and "spiritual" and would like to find a "spiritual outlet"
- Jane does not believe that she has a real chance at success

This represents the life formulation model in a nutshell. Let's take a closer look at some of its pluses.

Life Formulation Model Pluses

Some virtues of this life formulation model (and its accompanying Life Formulation Guide, which might eventually replace the DSM) include the following:

- It not only avoids the word "diagnosis" and the very idea of "diagnosis" (and essentially ends diagnosing), but it also avoids the word "psychological" and announces that a service provider is helping people in distress with their problems with living and not exclusively with their "psyche." Thus, for example, both "getting a job" and the "psychological consequences of not having a job" become legitimate areas of exploration. A helper could as legitimately work on "job skills" or "social skills" as work on any traditional "psychological" or "psychotherapeutic" issue.
- It doesn't conflate or confuse the person's concerns with the provider's concerns. Jane may not be concerned about her lack of sleep, her drinking, her cutting, or her eating habits, but her service provider may well be. This model allows both sorts of concerns to find a place in the conversation and a way to get both sorts of concerns communicated to third parties.
- It allows for conversations about, and reporting on, both "causes" (like suspected sexual abuse) and "treatment recommendations" (like, for example, cognitive work on self-esteem or behavioral work on stopping the cutting). No two providers might look at "causes" or "treatment recommendations" in the same way, but the life formulation model at least has built-in places for both to appear. "Causes" can appear in both "inferred challenges" and "provider's concerns," and "treatment" has a dedicated home in "provider's recommendations" (with the pseudo-medical word "treatment" studiously avoided).
- Some items could "auto-fill." If, for example, it is generally accepted that everyone should have a complete medical workup to see if the concerns presented are organic or biological in nature—to see, that is, if any "real" disease or medical condition is present—then one "standard recommendation" that could "auto-fill" would be "It is suggested that Jane have a complete medical workup."
  Likewise, if it is generally accepted that it is good to have someone to talk to about things, then the recommendation that "Jane should have

the chance to talk in an ongoing way with a service provider" might auto-fill. This latter point might seem obvious and go without saying, yet in the pseudo-medical model that we are disputing, it is not at all clear that "talking to someone" is seen as valuable, not when chemicals can be dispensed in a minute and save psychiatrists so much time and idle chit-chat. If we believe that "talking to someone" matters, it should be regularly included in our recommendations.

- It allows for an interesting "tag" system of reporting. This is an important point. When you search for something on the Internet you introduce certain words or "tags" that help you find what you are looking for, say "solar system," "planet," and "rings" if you are looking for a planet with rings. This gets you to "Saturn."

Tags are not labels but instead are our attempts to partially describe an entity. You can partially describe a thing in a "list sort of way" by identifying its parts: legs, head, tail, and so on (this is "defining by denotation"). You can also partially describe a thing in an "idea sort of way" through the use of concepts: a horse is a carbon-based living creature descended from some now extinct other carbon-based living creatures (this is "defining by connotation").

Such describing and defining is always incomplete, imperfect, and more arbitrary than we would like to admit. We know from philosophers of language like Wittgenstein that every abstract word (say "war" or "love") has no real definition but rather a huge range of meanings and colorations. Maybe World War II is the exemplary or paradigmatic instance of "war," but it is not meaningless or inappropriate to talk about "the war between the sexes" or "corporate warfare." The same is true of words like ego, dysfunction, abuse, or any other abstract word that can be used to describe human beings, human behaviors, and human situations.

Tags merely help describe: they do not amount to a "diagnosis," and they do not pretend to present an exhaustive, complete, or even adequate picture of a life. That is a good thing, because we should be tired by now of all that pretension. In Jane's case, you could report on Jane by providing some number of items in the six categories—say five items per category—and produce a one-page report that is thirty lines in length. That is one kind of "description of Jane's situation." But you could also choose from among those various items and select some number of tags—let's say seven—that together provide a kind of snapshot of Jane's current reality.

For example, one provider might choose as her seven tags for Jane and her situation "strict and punitive family dynamics," "low self-esteem coupled with high expectations," "adolescence," "self-starvation," "sadness," "excessive drinking," and "cutting." Naturally, each of these tags could come as a number rather than as words, if that was wanted. This snapshot would in no way provide a complete picture of Jane's current reality, but it would do a more sensible and humane job than labeling Jane with a pseudo-medical "clinical depression" diagnosis and some additional "adjustment disorder" or "personality disorder" diagnosis.

What might this tag system sound like in practice? For one person, and according to one service provider, the seven tags might be "sad," "unemployed," "mid-life crisis," "recently divorced, ""health issues," "'addicted' to porn," "no goals or aspirations." For another person, and according to another service provider, the seven tags might be, "traumatic childhood," "issues with food," "dramatic relationships," "spiritual seeker," "creatively unfulfilled," "uninspiring day job," "lives in 'chaos and confusion.'" These snapshots could be created around any agreed-upon number of tags. The more tags, the more cumbersome the system but also the more complete the snapshot.

If you decide to set the bar as, "We need one word like 'depression' to capture everything that we need to know about a person's distress and his or her current situation," a tag system does not reach that absurd height. But if you decide to set the bar differently as, "We need a way of communicating a snapshot of a person's reality that includes some important features of a person's life and aims a helper in the direction of helping," a tag system would meet that threshold beautifully.

- This model would "force" a service provider to inquire about Jane's actual concerns; learn about Jane's actual circumstances; acquire a picture of Jane's behaviors, thoughts, and feelings; come to some conclusions about Jane's situation; and offer up some recommendations as to what might help. This would naturally improve service. Service providers would become smarter about human nature and about human challenges by virtue of having to think about how "cause and effect" operates in the lives of real people and having to consider what actually works to reduce distress. This model stretches and tests the practitioner in a useful way.

To be clear, as we are not always so clear about this, this life formulation model is not an alternative system *of* diagnosis but an alternative system *to* diagnosis. It allows providers to chat with one another, either through summary reports or the tag system, and if it were widely accepted, it would force those entities that believe they need diagnoses (like, for example, the courts) to begin to change their mind. The courts and other institutions would be forced to accept that "hearing voices," for example, is a reportable thing but does not lead to some made-up diagnostic label like "schizophrenia." It would serve our vital communications needs and at the same time it would act as an agent of change.

No doubt other alternative systems to diagnosis can be dreamed up and one or another of them might provide even more pluses than this life formulation model. But this is a good start, I think; it could be enacted right now; and were it enacted, it would revolutionize how helpers think about and care for the people who come to them in difficulty and distress.

Technological Support

Imagine that a sophisticated software program were available to aid a practitioner using the life formulation model. Let's call this software "life formulation software" and imagine what it might do and how it might help.

To begin with, you would be able to pick one category or any number of categories called "orientations." One might be your personal orientation, which would be a customized orientation that you create. You could also pick any number of the many orientations that currently exist: a DSM orientation, an ICD orientation, a psychoanalytic orientation, a Jungian orientation, a systems orientation, an existential orientation, a psychological formulation orientation, a biological orientation, etc.

As you worked with a person in distress and entered information, that information would automatically be "digested" by the software in each of your chosen orientations, so that, for example, you would get a message (that of course you might choose to entirely ignore) that the threshold had been reached for a DSM or ICD diagnosis. In this way, you could be kept up-to-date about the labels being generated as you added information, and you would have at hand a Jungian vision of your client's presentation, or a DSM vision, an ICD vision, a psychoanalytic vision, and so on.

You would enter running information in the seven categories: 1) the person's expressed concerns; 2) the person's circumstances of note; 3) the person's behavioral and emotional considerations; 4) the person's goals and life purposes (a category I would like to see included); 5) the person's challenges as inferred by the provider; 6) the provider's concerns; and 7) the provider's recommendations. As you entered information, not only proposed "diagnoses" would appear, but also proposed tactics and strategies. For example, an alert might appear with the message "psychological formulation alert: check in on the possibility of childhood trauma," "Jungian alert: archetype of the gambler present," or "CBT alert: systematic desensitization suggested for fear of flying phobia."

For example, if you input "Marcia lost her sister to breast cancer when her sister was thirty-five and Marcia was thirty-nine," the DSM orientation would take in that information and likely consider it irrelevant; the existential orientation would take it in and "wonder aloud" if perhaps that event had provoked a meaning crisis; the CBT orientation would "wonder aloud" if any new language around mortality had entered

Marcia's internal vocabulary and, as a result, produced new anxiety in her; and so on. This would be done effortlessly, at the speed of computing, and the practitioner would either get that information as running commentary, in the margins, as it were, or get it when requested (for example, "Please tell me where we are now, existentially speaking").

The program could pop up all sorts of important notifications. For example, as you input the information that the person you are seeing is a male originally from the Caribbean living in London, it could pop up the announcement that males from the Caribbean living in London are x times more likely than the general population to receive a label of schizophrenia or y times more likely than the general population to be diagnosed with clinical depression. If you didn't want information of this sort to pop up, you could shut off this function; and you could also program the system so that it only popped up certain kinds of notifications.

Pop-up boxes might also appear that contrasted the views of the various orientations. For example, if you were to input the information that John "hears voices," a "compare and contrast" box might pop up with the following sort of information: "In the biological model, auditory hallucinations are considered possible symptoms of the following conditions and diseases; in the DSM model, auditory hallucinations are considered 'symptoms' of 'schizophrenia'; and in the psychological formulation model, hearing voices is considered one predictable response to stress, especially if the service user has a history of significant trauma."

Using software of this sort would also allow for regular updating of the different orientations. If the programmers of the psychoanalytic track or the CBT track wanted to make some changes based on new empirical evidence—wanted to include a new tactic to help with fear of flying or stopping smoking or "sadness reduction"—they could update "their portion of the program" and provide the practitioner with the most up-to-date information in their domain. In this way the practitioner would possess the best (or at least the latest) tactics, strategies, and methods from each domain, including the medical domains of brain diseases and neurological problems.

This "software support" beautifully serves the life formulation model and enhances its benefits. Its running commentary paints a clear picture that there is no agreement as to how to conceptualize these matters; it honors disagreement rather than fumbling us towards unjustified, artificial agreement; it reminds us that human beings can and must be viewed through multiple lenses. A human experience specialist using a life formulation model and its adjunctive, supportive software would be helped to understand and describe the reality of the person sitting across from her in multiple ways—in ways that might not interest her, like a DSM or ICD way, but also in ways that might interest her tremendously, including according to her own idiosyncratic orientation.

This idea of software support may prove fanciful: for one thing, most of the orientations in question probably aren't coherent or consistent enough to be programmed. Is there any such thing as a coherent, consistent Jungian, Freudian, cognitive-behavioral, or existential orientation? How could one program in a "psychological formulation" orientation or a "problems in living" orientation? On the other hand, some useful software support might indeed prove possible. There is no reason to suppose that we can't create a program that pops up an anxiety management tactic, a community resource, a cognitive-behavioral strategy, or an emotional healing technique right at the appropriate moment when a human experience specialist might want it, maybe before, during, or after a session.

This life formulation model, whether software supported or not, would go a long way toward providing a human experience specialist, or any practitioner looking to free herself from the DSM model or some other model, both with a conceptual framework that honors the richness of life and the naturalness of distress and an organizational scheme that allows her to report in an honest way on a sufferer's experience. In one sense, no such model is needed: the essence of our task is to lean forward and collaborate, not to report on our efforts. But a model that by its very nature disputes the DSM, that helps a practitioner ask the right questions, and that distinguishes her concerns from her client's concerns might well prove extremely valuable.

Some practitioners who are unhappy with the DSM model are nevertheless still looking for alternate methods *of* diagnosing: they are still attached to the idea of "diagnostic categories" that make reporting (and payment) easy and that allow them to continue to appear like "experts who diagnose and treat." That is a mistaken idea and a mistaken ideal for all the reasons we've been discussing. What are needed aren't alternative methods *of* diagnosing but excellent alternatives *to* diagnosis. We must stop "diagnosing" nonexistent "mental disorders" and instead find ways of talking sensibly about the problems of living that human beings experience. The life formulation model is one such sensible model.

18

The Brooklyn Project

Before I explain what I see as twenty keys to a mental health revolution, I want to describe a wide-ranging research project that would support such a revolution. This research project need not predate the revolution; it wouldn't be wise to wait on the revolution until research results came in. After all, research about being human, as opposed to research in the hard sciences, is highly overrated and probably shouldn't be called research at all. Greek and Roman philosophers knew a lot about being human without the benefit of any research. Indeed, it is not at all clear that we functionally know more now than we did then, when Aristotle, Plato, Socrates, Democritus, Heraclitus, Epicurus, Cicero, Aristophanes, Euclid, Euripides, and friends engaged in that wide-ranging thinking called "natural philosophy."

If learning about the research I have in mind doesn't interest you, please skip this chapter. But I think it is interesting in its own right, since its description sheds additional light on the issues we've been discussing. As I grew up in Brooklyn, and as the name I've picked is suggestive of another rather large, important project, the Manhattan Project, I've decided to call this research project the Brooklyn Project. The Brooklyn Project could be carried out worldwide at many collaborating institutions, at one particular academic institution, or at a governmental institute parallel to the National Institute of Mental Health. Its physical location and auspices would matter considerably less than the quality, heart, and courage of the researchers involved.

Its overarching goal would not be to arrive at perfect answers or even decent answers to the questions researchers posed but for the first time to look critically at what we claim to know about being human. This is an impossible, messy goal that reverses the academic trend of narrowly looking at "psychology," "anthropology," "sociology," and so on, and takes as its evidence and its interests everything, absolutely everything, just as the Greek and Roman natural philosophers did. It might well not even call itself a research project, as research is a word that suggests science and knowing. Maybe it would describe itself as a worldwide super-brainstorming session about being human.

Brilliant people would be needed for this. Right now many of those brilliant people go into the hard sciences. We understand why. But perhaps some disaffected hard scientists who have seen the limits of science and would like to do some fascinating blue-sky thinking will come aboard and join top-notch youngsters who intuit that the Brooklyn Project might be much more interesting—and valuable—than software engineering or particle physics. Lawyers, doctors, businesspeople, poets, and other disaffected souls who, never previously having found a place to deeply think, might join them too.

Let us remember that there is an agenda here, in addition to better understanding what it means to be human. That is to interrogate and ultimately to overthrow the current mental health establishment model of "diagnosing" and "treating." The primary activity of the Brooklyn Project would be to step right into the forefront of the battle being waged against current constructs. It is first of all asking the question, "What is it exactly that psychiatry does?" and second of all demanding, "Let us put the whole field of psychology under a microscope." It would look closely at all of the issues we've discussed so far: what we mean by normal and abnormal, what we mean by cause and effect in human affairs, what actually helps reduce emotional distress and who should be tasked with helping the distressed, what makes for better mental health institutions and therapeutic communities, and so on.

That is, the Brooklyn Project is a mental health project. It is looking at everything human not so as to create some sort of new encyclopedia of humanness but so as to come up with recommendations about what needs to change in current mental health practices and what better mental health practices might look like. While the National Institute of Mental Health is looking at "the biological bases of mental illness," the wild bunch at the Brooklyn Project would be throwing everything about "mental health" into question for the sake of arriving at more understanding and best practices. Its agenda is not the accumulation of knowledge but the creation of a whole new way of looking at "mental health."

Here are some of the sorts of issues that might occupy folks at the Brooklyn Project:

1. If we want to start fresh and do a better job of conceptualizing "mental health" and "mental disorders" so as to provide more help to sufferers, what sort of research agenda might we set? First, what do we mean by "research"

in this context? Do we mean experiments involving human beings? Do we mean white coat science? Do we mean observation and empiricism? Do we mean statistical analysis? Do we mean thought experiments, as in theoretical physics? Do we mean rounding up anecdotal evidence, say from "mental health patients"? Do we mean "Just thinking"? As a corollary question, might graduate students who are currently obliged to do research be allowed to tackle large "meta questions," even if those efforts look more like natural philosophy than science? What is the "right way" or "right ways" to "research" what it means to be human?

2. How might we conceptualize the task of rethinking mental health if research turns out to be out of the question? How, for example, could we research the nature of the original endowment with which each individual arrives in the world (what I have elsewhere called "original personality")? Can this be researched or is research here out of the question? How could we research the amount of sadness generated by a stray cloud passing in front of the sun twenty years ago in the life of a given individual? Isn't research about such things completely impossible? How could we research what we mean by "normal" and "abnormal"? What if much of what we need to know can't be researched? What, if any, are the alternatives to scientific research, and by what criteria would we want to judge the soundness, reliability, or usefulness of each of these alternative approaches?

3. What various definitions of "mental health" might be proposed? How might we characterize the underlying idea of each definition? If a given definition of mental health rested on some other construct like "good coping skills," "resilience," "high functioning in society," "absence of undue emotional distress," or "self-report of contentment," what is our rationale for choosing that underlying construct rather than a competing one? Who would decide which definition of "mental health" ought to be used and by what authority would that entity get to make such a decision? As a corollary question, what category of person should be considered "expert" in the matter of defining "mental health," given the poor record of current and past putative experts? Given that the very idea of "mental health" is up for grabs, who should be authorized to grab it?

4. What are the various possible relationships between "mental health" and "emotional distress"? For example, is it reasonable to suppose that a person could be mentally healthy but also emotionally distressed? Surely it is. Is it reasonable to suppose that a person could be mentally unhealthy, whatever that phrase might mean, and also not mentally distressed at all? For example, might not a mentally healthy person be considerably distressed by the famine affecting his society and a mentally unhealthy person experience no distress as he commits a murder? If the relationship between "mental health" and "emotional distress" isn't straightforward and if we aren't entitled to say that the presence of emotional distress means the absence of mental health, what are various ways that we might conceptualize the relationship between the two? To put the question differently, is there any "amount"

of emotional distress the presence of which "generates" the label of "mentally unhealthy" or "mentally disordered"? If the answer is no, are we saying that "emotional distress" and "mental health" are unconnected, or are we saying that they are connected but in complicated and even seemingly paradoxical ways?

5. What are the current "psychological models of distress" (like, for example, the Freudian model), "mental disorder models of distress" (like, for example, the DSM model), and "social and political models of distress" (say, for example, the Marxist model)? How do we judge their strengths and weaknesses? And how do we tease out what we want a knowledgeable service provider to know from these models? What do we want to "do" with all these existing models? At least get them listed, described, and organized? As a corollary idea, what constructs or concepts within a given psychological model are strong, true, or sensible? Even if a given theory, vision, or set of opinions is not strong in its aggregate, how might we judge if a given idea within it is useful? For example, might the idea of a "midlife crisis" be a useful concept irrespective of whether or not any other Jungian ideas are useful or true? How can we judge the strength, truth, or importance of the countless concepts that have already been generated?

6. To what extent do we currently rely on self-reports to "diagnose mental disorders," and if that reliance is very high (or even total), on what else might we rely? What do we rely on in medicine to make diagnoses and to what extent is any of that apparatus currently available or logically applicable when it comes to "mental distress" or "mental disorder"? If what we are talking about has little or nothing to do with "the brain" and everything to do with "the mind," on what should we rely in addition to or separate from self-reports from the individual? As a corollary idea, if we designate someone as entitled to "diagnose mental disorders," what ought we demand that he or she rely on separate from or in addition to the self-report of the individual? If he or she says, "I observed the individual," by what criteria shall we judge that what was observed amounted to a "mental disorder" and not something else? If he or she says, "I tested the individual," by what criteria shall we judge the appropriateness or soundness of the test itself given the way that psychological tests are constructed and given that they are self-reports. To put this another way, how do we "test" for what ails a person—especially if what ails a person is life?

7. How might we conceptualize an individual's contribution to the maintenance of his or her emotional distress? If, for example, an individual agrees that she would feel less sad if she did x but is reluctant to do x, how might we conceptualize that reluctance? Might we say, for example, that it is hard to make a change, even a desired one, that there are "unconscious reasons for her reluctance," that "not rocking the boat is more important to her than reducing her sadness," and so on? What (presumably very many) hypotheses might we generate as to why people do not do what they know to do to reduce their mental

distress or improve their lives? Second, how can we come to know which hypotheses are true so that we could arm helpers with tactics for dealing with this disinterest in or lack of cooperation? As a corollary idea, how might we gauge or measure an individual's contribution to the maintenance of his or her emotional distress? How can we know when and to what extent an individual is participating in the maintenance of his or her distress? To say this differently, if our goal is to help, how do we factor in the extent to which the people we intend to help are often not very helpful?

8. What do we take "behavior" to stand for or count for? What sort of marker is bed-wetting, "excessive" hand washing, "alcoholic" drinking, or a suicide gesture? What are the arguments for linking any given behavior to a construct called a "mental disorder" or a "mental disease"? If we claim that it is some single necessary linkage, like "lack of control," how do we know if the individual lacks that control or prefers not to exert that control? If an individual can go from "drinking alcoholically" one day to "entering recovery" the next, what did we mean by "lack of control" when and if we used it as a criterion for labeling? What, if any, are the ways that we can get at a true or accurate picture of the relationship between observed behavior and the generating cause or causes of that behavior? If we can't really know the linkage between "the mind" and "behavior," what should we take observable behavior to mean?

9. To continue on this theme, how should we conceptualize the differences between or the relationships between a behavior and an inner state? Tossing aside the book you're reading is a behavior. Tossing it aside because it bores you or because it angers you reflects an inner state of mind, tossing it aside because it has become electrified is a biological reflex, tossing it aside because a policeman orders you to toss it aside reflects a social interaction, and so on. Tossing the book aside is an "observable behavior," but what it means is not known simply by observing such an action out of its human context. How can we conceptualize the task of relating observable behavior to the "causes" or "sources" of that behavior?

10. How do we retain the sense that a human being is involved here? Humanistic psychology, person-centered psychology, and existential psychology, to name a few "psychological orientations," explicitly state that the individual is a member of a certain species with certain human desires and challenges, that he or she must be consulted, respected, and understood, and that a "real person" is different from a "patient." Other orientations take different stances, and in the current "medical model," we have lost the person almost entirely. How might a human being's "individuality and instrumentality" be conceptualized, do we know enough to do that conceptualizing, and if we don't know enough, where should we err? On the side of "acting as if" the individual is a person, a collection of dynamic forces, a symptom generator, or something else? How might we tease apart "the place of the person" in relation to the provision of mental health services, with an eye to generating respect and compassion for the individual in question?

11. In line with the above, what shall we call a person who walks into the office of a "mental health service provider"? Since there are many compelling reasons not to call that person a "patient," shall we call that person a "client," as that is the other term most often used in this context? Is there a better word to use than "patient" or "client," and what are the arguments for that better word or those better words? In some contexts we call a person a customer (when she enters a store), in some a client (when she hires a lawyer), in some a patient (when she sees her dentist), in some a parishioner (when she sits with her priest), in some a student (when she takes a class), and so on. What is the relationship with a mental health provider most like, and if it is different from all of the above, do we need a new word to communicate that difference? (A full discussion of this issue can be found in chapter 5.)

12. What will a "new mental health service provider" provide? If it is wise to repudiate the DSM "medical catalogue" approach, as I believe it is, and if we come to see that it is not appropriate to act as if the interaction between client and provider is the "diagnosing and treating of mental disorders," what will a person currently called a "psychotherapist" or some new provider be doing or providing? Will his or her "talk" not need to change at all in some cases? Has he or she perhaps been simply providing "wise counsel" all along and never really "diagnosing and treating mental disorders" and therefore not need to change his or her tactics? On the other hand, will some providers need to completely overhaul what they do, insofar as they were operating from and invested in the "medical catalogue" model? As a corollary idea, what should the state claim to be sanctioning and what position should it take with respect to "standards of care"? If it acts as if there are "mental disorders to be diagnosed and treated" and demands that its licensed or certified professionals play along with this idea even if in their office they simply offer wise counsel, should this shadow game end? If so, what would the fallout be, for example, in the courts? What do we want providers to provide, and how can we get society aligned with what may prove to be completely new standards of care?

13. If it turns out that something like a "wise counsel" model is the most appropriate model for service provision, how do we train "wise counselors" (providers I have dubbed human experience specialists), how do we change curricula to reflect our new understanding about the logic and content of courses like "introduction to abnormal psychology" or "understanding the DSM," and how do we distinguish between "coaching" and "psychotherapy"? In short, how do we conceptualize the change in the naming and training of "mental health service providers" to reflect the changes that might be wanted? What do we do "with" or "about" existing psychiatrists, psychologists, marriage and family therapists, clinical social workers, and other "mental health service providers"? Do we allow them to continue on "as is" even if the game has changed? Do we demand that they make certain changes in their outlook and their practices, changes that they must somehow "prove"

have occurred (for example, through continuing education classes)? If, for example, it becomes common wisdom and general understanding that there is no "mental disorder of depression," can we allow mental health service providers to keep "diagnosing and treating depression"? What are our options in this regard?

14. Whether or not we ever understand what is really going on in the minds of people, we nevertheless want to be of aid to people seeking help with their emotional distress. Given that, what helps? How shall we research the "best helping methods" given that we may well not be talking about organic problems but reactions to life challenges? How can we tease out the relationships between a given problem (say, despair or intense anxiety) and the best, most logical, or most appropriate "treatment methods" or "helping methods"? What do we take "this really works" to mean in this context: that a "symptom is removed," that a person's life is radically changed for the better, that the presenting problem (like despair) still remains but the individual can tolerate it better, and so on? We need a wide-ranging exploration of what "help" means in a human context, which "help" helps the most, and which "help" we ought to offer according to which problem is presented. (For example, is the same "help" best for despair, anxiety, addictive behaviors, etc.?)

15. What might be the rationale for a given helping strategy or tactic? What is the legitimacy of that rationale? Can we perhaps employ strategies without knowing their rationale or without granting the legitimacy of that rationale if individuals report that the strategy has helped them? For example, should we grant dream interpretation a place at the helping table even if there is no proof that "dreams are the royal road to the unconscious" and even if the practitioner has no rationale at all for using it except to say, "I know it helps"? Is a self-report of reduced emotional distress or some other self-report of ratification on a client's part "enough" to validate helping methods, given what we know about the placebo effect? Is a self-report of success the only validation necessary, or might there be other methods or measures? How might the matter of "How do we know what helps?" be conceptualized?

16. What is cause and what is effect? When, for example, we see a certain pattern in a brain scan, how should we go about deciding whether the individual's despair caused that brain look or whether that brain look is actually telling us anything about the cause of his or her despair? Is our sleeplessness a cause of our anxiety or is our anxiety a cause of our sleeplessness? What is cause and what is effect, what is chicken and what is egg? How can complicated causal chains in human affairs be examined or understood, and how can this problem be best articulated and addressed? If perhaps we can't ever know what is cause and what is effect, what helping strategies might we nevertheless employ in the absence of that knowledge? Is there "best help" to provide if you do know the cause or causes of the distress and different "best help" to provide if you can't know the cause or causes of the distress?

17. What do we mean by "reducing emotional distress" or "improving our mental health"? As an important corollary idea, is "feeling better" always the highest good? For example, if a lobotomy would reduce or eliminate your emotional distress but also make you a zombie, surely that is too high a price to pay for "feeling better." What if a chemical can help you feel better in some senses and worse in other senses? How can we measure the "net benefits" of a chemical or a strategy when it produces both positives and negatives? What are the "right" or appropriate prices to pay for feeling better? Is "feeling better" even the goal? How can these matters be conceptualized?

18. Given the variety of stakeholders, the history and customs of the trade, and the fact that the welfare and emotional health of hundreds of millions of human beings worldwide will be affected by any changes to the model and the system (including all the people taking "medication" for what may no longer be seen as "medical disorders or diseases"), how should we handle this moment and determine who takes responsibility? If a certain shift turns out to be clearly desirable, should it be a bottom-up shift (for example, with new human experience specialists hanging out their shingles, with ad campaigns plastered on the sides of buses, and so on), a top-down shift (for example, with the empaneling of a governmental "blue ribbon panel" made up of system insiders but also of system outsiders), or both? If conclusions are reached and action steps proposed, how can those action steps be implemented in the real world?

It is easier to understand the workings of the universe than the workings of a person. With human beings, there is much that is strictly unknowable. We can't know if a person is born with a particular original personality and with a particular blueprint for development. We can't know enough about the virtually infinite number of links in the causal chain that produces a feeling or a behavior. We can't know whether a person is visited by emotional distress or invites that visitation. The list of what we can never know about human beings is very long and includes what is most important to know.

But we also don't know if we can't perhaps do a much better job—a really improved job—of knowing. The folks at The Brooklyn Project would give that a try. They would shake their heads at the absurdity of the task and the impossibility of success and then roll up their sleeves and see what new understanding is possible. The Manhattan Project arose because of the astounding threat that Hitler posed. Our current threat is also unprecedented: the threat to our children, that virtually all of them will find themselves with a mental disorder diagnosis and on a regimen of powerful chemicals, and the threat to everyone that our unchallenged "epidemic of emotional distress" is causing. A Brooklyn Project might help.

19

Twenty Keys to a Mental Health Revolution

Let me summarize the points I've made in the previous eighteen chapters, consolidate my ideas, and point us in the direction of a better future for mental health service provision and individual mental health. Here is what I would like to see:

1. I want the very ideas of "mental disorder" and "mental disease" questioned and a new picture painted of distress occurring as a result of being human and because of problems in living and not because of mental viruses and chemical imbalances. We would drop the game of "diagnosing" and "treating" and ask ourselves, "What makes human beings human, and what can we do to help people who are suffering?"

2. If this shift can be made from "mental disorder" to "problems of living," then we might be able to also make a change in our thinking from "medications used to treat mental illness" to "chemicals with effects that may or may not produce an effect you want to handle one of your problems with living." I would want fewer human beings on these chemicals, especially far fewer children.

3. I would want all that we do not know much more honored so that we can finally really get at, insofar as it is possible to do so, cause and effect in human matters and a better sense of what actually helps. There would also need to be a way of speaking about "all that we don't know" that prevents the mental health establishment from retorting, "Look, you say that you don't know, and we say that we do know, so we win!" One of the tremendous challenges in moving forward is finding language that allows us to announce that there is a lot that we do not know without allowing that not knowing to become a decisive factor in dismissing reform initiatives.

4. I would want us to carefully avoid a proliferation of new manuals, catalogues, lists, menus, and other systems that might be thought to be better than the DSM method but that do not do the real (and hard and maybe impossible) work required of a truly better manual. For example, some new "manual of concerns" (which is being floated as

an idea) would prove no improvement, since the same faulty transaction as presently occurs would continue. You come in and say that you are sad. I look up your concern in my manual of concerns, find it, and agree, "You are concerned that you are sad." This isn't an improved transaction.

In this transaction we still do not have a hint of cause and effect or "what helps" on the table. I have only mirrored or parroted what you have told me. A genuinely improved manual, if it is even possible to create one, would need to do a real and sophisticated job of linking up varieties of cause and effect, the patterns produced by this amazing variety, and what then helps, either with regard to one particular "pattern" or generically, rather than just providing some list of "concerns" or "problems."

5. I would want us to think through how institutions that currently exist might be improved and how different institutions—for example, therapeutic communities of care—might be supported. The current institutional approach has mainly to do with society's need to warehouse dangerous and difficult people and keep society safe from and segregated from folks who, for example, are hearing voices or threatening to kill themselves.

    In the current model (like in all prison models) the number one goal is not "treatment" (or, in prison jargon, "rehabilitation") but the management of difficult persons. Some or perhaps many members of the institution may actually want to help, but the institution as a whole is predicated on one commandment: "Control the inmates and keep the guards safe." Naturally, we would expect coercive methods to flourish in institutions with this mandate just as we would expect them to flourish in prisons, and this is exactly what we see. I would want us to look at all this and make changes.

6. I want to create a simple, easy-to-articulate, but also accurate snapshot of what is currently going on so that we might know what we want to change and where we want to go. Here is one example of what such a simple snapshot might look like. I think that it is fair to say that the current mental health establishment operates in the following five ways:

    There is an atheoretical, profit-driven DSM-based diagnostic and treatment model that is the "thing" in contrast to which alternatives are most wanted. In this DSM model, where mental disorders are created in a room by folks sitting around a table, the putative goals are symptom relief, mood alteration, behavior change, and so on, achieved primarily through chemical intervention. The sufferer's "symptoms" are combined into a "symptom picture" and labeled as a certain "mental disorder." Then the "appropriate medication" is prescribed as the only treatment or else with some adjunctive "talk therapy" added.

    There is no particular interest taken in knowing what is "causing" the distress; no particular interest taken in understanding the person's circumstances, pressures, economic class, and so on; and no rationale offered for the treatments proposed except to say, "We are doing a sort of medicine." This is the main thrust of current mental health service provision, backed staunchly by psychiatrists, drug companies, and anyone else able to profit from an easy-to-use catalogue of labels.

There are also many theory-based diagnostic and treatment models. Many practitioners, such as psychotherapists, use this model (without, however, always announcing in an aboveboard way that this is indeed what they are doing). In this model, a mental health professional relies on some perhaps coherent or perhaps incoherent set of ideas, loosely called a theory, that provide a rationale for naming causes and effects (diagnosing) and for proposing a set of tactics, strategies, or methods called "treatments." All of the following are examples of one or another "theory-based diagnostic and treatment model":

- "Your faulty cognitions are causing your emotional distress, and we are going to work on creating some thought substitutes for those faulty cognitions (cognitive theory and cognitive treatment)."
- "Because of your early childhood experiences, you failed to form a strong, healthy bond with yourself, and now we are going to work on improving your self-relationship (self-psychology attachment theory and self-psychology treatment)."
- "Because your id impulses are so strong, your punitive super-ego is working overtime and treating you very harshly. We need to replace those id impulses with a better functioning ego, and we'll begin with some dream analysis (Freudian theory and Freudian treatment).
- "Your mind is causing your suffering, and I have an ancient, time-honored seven-fold path to propose to you as a way for you to get a grip on your mind and relieve your suffering. Key to this effort is daily meditation (Buddhist theory and Buddhist treatment)."
- "We all create stories, and then not only do we live those stories, but we tend to be held hostage by them. Let's work on rewriting your story (narrative therapy and narrative treatment).

All of the many pseudo-theories and pseudo-systems extant—and there are scores of them, from Jungian theory to personality trait theory, from existential theory to occult theories—provide the helper with a picture of how to conceptualize what is wrong (e.g., faulty thinking) and what helps (e.g., daily meditation). Providing a particular form of help is then rationalized or justified on the basis of a particular picture of what causes human suffering.

Third is a client-centered approach, which is probably what most therapists actually do in practice. A helper asks a person who comes in, "What's going on?", the helper listens, and drawing from his or her experiences and thoughts about life asks further questions, makes suggestions, proposes tactics, and so on. The essential quality of this approach is that two human beings are sitting across from one another and chatting seriously.

At one extreme, the helper keeps "returning the work" to the sufferer by repeatedly asking, "What do you think about what you just said?" or "And how did that make you feel?" Most client-centered helpers, however, also offer advice, teach, suggest, and make considerable use of themselves and what they know. In this model, which, depending on how it is held and practiced, can amount to a complete "no-diagnosis" model and is very much like what a human experience specialist might do, little or no "diagnosing" or labeling tends to go on.

Fourth is the "pure biology" or "pure science" approach, in which a hunt is conducted for "the biological bases of mental disease." This is the current approach of, for example, the National Institute of Mental Health. There are grave problems with this approach: directionality issues (what causes what—for example, does sadness change the brain or does a brain malfunction cause the sadness?), definitional and theoretical issues (what are the diseases for which biological bases are being hunted?—If, for example, there is no such "disease" as "depression" or "schizophrenia," what exactly is a biological researcher hunting for?), etc. Given these and many similar problems, it is not at all clear that science is actually being conducted here, even though the researchers may be trained "hard" scientists.

Fifth are all the institutional approaches, from outpatient group work under the auspices of an HMO to court-referred drinking driver programs to social worker caseloads to locked ward for-profit mental institutions to forensic psychology and court-related pronouncements on mental health and so on.

To say this all simply, we need a sensible way of describing what currently goes on, and the following is one plausible way. What currently goes on has five faces to it: 1) a psychiatric/pseudo-medical DSM approach; 2) a pseudo-theory-based psychotherapy approach; 3) a client-centered psychotherapy approach; 4) a biological hunt approach; and 5) generally coercive institutional approaches. With some additions, this is rather the whole landscape of current mental health service provision practices.

7. We would want to know what additional methods, systems, constructs, and institutions already exist in addition to the five I just described. Others do indeed currently exist—for example, a team approach with "flying teams" that come to your door, like the Finnish Open Dialogue method I described in chapter 14, and the "communities of care" approach, where, for example, you as a sufferer come to work on a farm and live in a therapeutic community. Many "alternate approaches" are already out there—we should create a robust menu of these already-existing alternatives, maybe to include everything from pastoral counseling to AA to life coaching. If what we are looking at are indeed "problems in living" and not "mental disorders," then whatever helps

a sufferer better deal with his or her problems ought to have a place on this menu of already-existing resources.

8. I would want us to dream up many new alternatives. There might be alternatives to the current diagnostic approach, alternatives to the theory-driven approach, alternatives to the client-centered approach, alternatives to the biological hunt approach, alternative institutional approaches, and other alternatives that do not fit into any of these five categories. For example, here are three alternative approaches that both resemble and are different from what is currently available:

A "patterns" model that might sound something like, "You say that you are having trouble with anxiety. There look to be some patterns in the lives of people with anxiety, both in terms of what is provoking the anxiety and in terms of what may help relieve the anxiety. I am not saying that we know what is 'causing' your anxiety and I am not saying that I know what can 'cure' your anxiety. But let me tell you a little bit about the patterns that we think we see, and you can tell me what seems to fit for you."

In this model, the mental health professional announces that she does indeed have a certain kind of expertise, an expertise in knowing about "patterns of distress formation and relief," so she is not so purely "client-centered" as the sort of helper who returns all the work to the sufferer. The question arises as to whether this model would "creep" in the direction of a catalogue or manual of "patterns"? It seems natural that such creep would occur. A second question then becomes, "Is this creep perhaps legitimate and worthy or is it a slide back toward labeling and 'diagnosing'?" These are the sorts of open questions we would want to ask about any alternative proposal.

A wrinkle on the client-centered approach might be a "dialogue approach." Dialogue has about it a sense of give and take, curiosity and engagement. If you are telling me a long, long story, we are not in dialogue. That is you in monologue. If you tell me something and I come back with a canned question, that is not dialogue. That is boilerplate. If, no matter what you say, I steer you back someplace, that is not dialogue. That is arm-wrestling. The fundamental quality of dialogue is that I am listening and that you are listening. If you are not listening, I am obliged to point that out. If I am not listening, you are obliged to point that out.

It is not at all hard to picture how an alternative model of helping, for example, one leading to the creation of that projected new helper, the human experience specialist, might grow out of the simple idea of dialogue. As we examine all possible alternatives, we would have no reason to scorn an alternative as too simple, too nontechnical, or too nonmedical. Let us get the alternatives on the table first and then, and only then, see what we like and what we don't like about each.

All sorts of new "helping models" might emerge, for example, a "skills building" model or a "new habits" model. A "skills building" model might be created around an idea promoted in certain recovery circles, where the acronym CHIME (connectedness, hope, identity, meaning, and empowerment) stands for five "key recovery practices." In this model, a sufferer would be told, "It's likely that working on these five skills will help you." Then work on those five skills would amount to the centerpiece focus of that model. Or a "new habits" model might be proposed, the argument being that what is most needed in the life of someone suffering are "new habits that help with the challenges of being human." Such a practitioner might even have a "menu of new habits" to share with the sufferer.

Countless alternatives might be proposed. If we weren't too quick to anoint any one new alternative as *the* alternative, there would prove no harm in having this list of alternatives grow really large. We might encounter new ways of thinking about psychological formulation; new models that focus on social justice and social constructivist concerns; new symptom-focused models that make clear what a symptom "is" ("That's likely a symptom of something going on. Let's try two things at once: let's try to ease the symptom and also see if we can figure out what's causing it"); new goal-oriented, quasi-coaching models; and new models premised in ways that we have not thought of before. No approach would be quickly ratified, but a mental health practitioner could look at this array of alternatives and say, "Hmm, that new dialogue method looks really interesting to me—I might just take it out for a spin!"

9. We need to get all of these alternatives, both those that currently exist and those that might be proposed, "in one place," maybe on a website run for the benefit of humanity. How these many alternatives could be presented "objectively" is a very difficult question to answer since so many of the words that are currently used (like "diagnosis," "treatment," etc.) are completely loaded. But let us imagine that this presentation issue isn't insurmountable. Implicit in the idea of inviting new alternatives to come forward is the idea that we would get to know about these new alternatives, think about them, chat about them, and so forth, so let us make that implicit idea explicit: gathering together and sharing existing models and new models are important tasks of the revolution.

10. We desperately need a clear picture of what actually helps. In fact, we already know about many things that help. We know that the warmth and humanness of the mental health service provider helps. There is tremendous evidence on that score. The warmer and more human the provider, the better the outcome. Doesn't it seem likely that teaching helps, that skill-building helps, that providing useful homework helps, that holding a sufferer accountable for taking action helps, that inquiring into what's going on helps, that providing basic information helps, that pointing the way to resources and making referrals help, that creating a spirit of cooperation and collaboration helps, that knowing something (for example, knowing what dozen tactics help reduce a person's experience of anxiety) helps, that the provider being calm helps, and so on?

It would be lovely for a really long list of what helps to be created—and better yet, it would be wonderful if a careful job could be done connecting up "what helps" with "when to use a given strategy." Don't we need a smart, sensible "guide to helping strategies and when to use them"? Are there better times to listen, better times to inquire, better times to interrupt, better times to instruct, better times to confront? Are there excellent helping strategies to tease out of the myriad theoretical approaches to psychotherapy, pulling, for example, three useful tactics out of Freudian practice, four useful tactics out of Jungian practice, five useful tactics out of cognitive-behavioral practice, and so on? Wouldn't such a guide, whatever its flaws and shortfalls, nevertheless go a long way toward arming helpers with an arsenal of helping strategies?

11. We need much better thinking, much more clarity, and a much more careful use of language overall, as I described in the last chapter on the Brooklyn Project. We need to stop using words like "normal" and "abnormal" if they mean nothing. We need to distinguish between medications and chemicals. We need to look carefully at the hideously empty definitions of "mental disorder" promulgated by the DSM-4 and now the DSM-5—definitions that have changed radically from one edition to the next for no other reason than to meet appropriate objections leveled at the definition of a "mental disorder" in the DSM-4. We need to stop creating ecumenical, completely meaningless umbrella "causes" for "mental disorders" by claiming, for example, that they are "biopsychosocial" in nature. Everything human is biopsychosocial in nature! We need more honesty and better thinking than that.

We need top thinkers, who perhaps currently shy away from the world of mental health as a too muddy, too soft, and too difficult a place in which to do real science, to inquire of themselves, "Yes, that would prove a truly difficult place, but isn't having a say about the future of the emotional health of our species more important than participating in the creation of a new phone or a new television?" We need strong, smart people who know a thing or two about being human to help foment and manage a revolution away from the current pseudo-medical approach to mental health, where even nonmedical folks like clinical psychologists are inveigling their way into prescribing "medications for mental illnesses." We need strong, smart people to begin to really help the billions of people who experience emotional distress and who might love to have some real help offered to them.

12. We could train, sanction, and legitimize a new category of helper, the human experience specialist, who would operate free of the baggage currently burdening psychotherapists, family therapists, clinical social workers, psychologists, psychiatrists, and other established mental health workers who, irrespective of what they actually believe, must act as if they believe in medical-sounding ideas and the current "mental disorder" labeling system.

13. We could, even in the absence of any agreement about what we meant by "mental health," affirm that certain life skills are good things and begin to teach them in our schools in addition to and alongside academic subjects. We could teach our children how to align their thoughts and their behaviors with their intentions, how to retain their individuality in a group setting, how to self-regulate and tolerate ambiguity and difference, how to seize meaning opportunities and make meaning investments, and so on. All of this could be taught.

14. For children and adults both, we could provide stress reduction techniques, anxiety management techniques, recovery techniques, and other helpful techniques as part of a nationwide and worldwide effort at preventative health care, since not a soul doubts that not being able to effectively handle stress, anxiety, addictive impulses, and other common human challenges lead inexorably to medical problems that come with substantial costs and that tax any health care system.

15. We could strive to reduce or eliminate those "mental health issues" attached to poverty by reducing or eliminating poverty. Anything that helps a person live a less painful life, like having a home rather than living on the streets, helps that person with his or her "mental health issues." A genuine effort to help the poorest among us would amount to a major societal mental health goal.

16. We could create and support institutions and communities of care, as described in chapter 14. These institutions could be run for profit and as businesses or as nonprofits or charities. They might be created strategically in conjunction with some other societal need or goal, like producing food, producing energy, recycling waste materials, and so on. Insofar as a given therapeutic community as a whole—a particular farm community, say, or recycling community—believed in the meaningfulness of the work it was doing, so too might the sufferers who arrived to join in that work, thus helping create new meaning opportunities for those suffering from chronic meaning problems.

17. We could launch all sorts of initiatives and public service advertising campaigns that in simple language and through clear messages underline the challenges that human beings face. These campaigns could offer suggestions as to how to handle those challenges. Spectacularly simple messages could begin to appear on the sides of buses and in between television shows, just as powerful anti-smoking messages currently do. Rather than focusing on one particular issue—domestic violence, say, or alcohol abuse or anxiety management—these campaigns would "step back" and announce that being human comes with predictable, painful challenges and that help is available.

18. We could educate our children about the demanding nature of life and the likelihood that they will experience difficulties. At the same time, we could sell them on humanistic values, encourage them not to let their personality become their destiny, and paint a clear, simple picture of value-based meaning making. These life lessons could be taught in schools, but since that is rather unlikely to happen,

teachers could point students to cyberspace resources and embrace cyber education as a great adjunctive tool to brick-and-mortar education.

19. We could communicate the fact that meaning is a psychological experience and that there are many different ways to acquire that psychological experience—that many sorts of meaning opportunities are available to human beings—and in this simple way help people better understand the work required of them to make life feel meaningful. We could communicate the opportunities available to reduce their existential pain.

20. We need a fundamental shift—nowadays typically called a "paradigm shift"—in our basic orientation away from the ideas of "mental disorder" and "mental disease" and toward a more rounded, sophisticated, and truer vision of what it means to be human, how life naturally produces distress, how our formed personality works to lock in that distress, and what helps to relieve that distress. We likewise need a new professional to help with human problems—a human experience specialist—someone who knows a lot more than just "psychology" and an awful lot about being human and negotiating life's challenges.

We need all these changes. We especially need them because our children are under siege. It is one thing for an adult to accept that his despair is a "mental disorder" that can be "treated" with a chemical. He is an adult, after all, and entitled to make that choice. It is another thing for a five-year-old to find himself on three or four psychiatric chemicals. There are many reasons why we require a mental health revolution but let's underline just one of these many: to spare the children. Do we want every single child labeled and treated as a mental patient just because a professional class can get away with playing a very profitable game?

20

The Future of Your Mental Health

If you are currently suffering, this book may not have spoken to you much except between the lines. It isn't a great help to be told that you are human and that you must deal with it. If you are in unyielding circumstances, it isn't wonderful to hear that your circumstances matter. It isn't much of a relief to learn that the first step of your journey is from "the mental disorder of depression" to ordinary despair or from "the mental illness of schizophrenia" to a complicated reality that includes the straightjacket of your formed personality and experiences, such as hearing voices. What have I really offered you?

I would say that I have offered you an opening. My offer is that you leave a table set with a feast of false views of your reality and second-rate answers to your challenges and decide, despite the overwhelming constraints put on you by your formed ways of being, to plot your own course. I would ask you to articulate your values and your principles and live a life full of purpose with a fiendish new talent for making personal meaning. Popping a pill no doubt sounds easier; that is your choice. The door I am inviting you to open leads through a gauntlet of cold water to a vast expanse of reality.

The problem you face is being human. If the problem really was some biological malfunction, that would be one thing. But it isn't. The problem is your personality; the problem is the causal chain that is your history; the problem is your circumstances; the problem is the way your pain manifests; the problem is the world as it is; the problem is your reality. It is a problem that never ends and is never resolved. Who are we trying to kid by not facing our destiny? There are evolutionary reasons for widespread denial, but even if that denial helps the species as a whole, it is unlikely that it helps you very much—not if you are suffering.

The instant we pat ourselves on the back that we have resolved one thing or made one thing better—finally created meaningful work, say, or had the great luck of meeting someone to love—then a cloud passes over the sun and we remember how many children are starving or how we will cease to exist in the blink of an eye or how much trouble we are having trying to quit smoking. Let us stop trying to live pain-free and live proudly instead. Our true goal is to try to reduce all the emotional distress that we can possibly reduce while at the same time sighing at the inevitable return of some portion of it.

If you are chronically poor, chronically in physical pain, chronically sad, chronically unable to realize your dreams, chronically unable to experience life as meaningful, that is really too much. Yet somehow you must soldier through life, even if you would really just as soon not bother. There is no good answer to this—a million beers are not the answer; voodoo is not the answer; shopping is not the answer; rage is not the answer. While there is no good answer, there is nevertheless a best answer. That is the way of pride, power, purpose, and inner peace that begins with a deep acceptance of the nature of being human.

Our personality forms around many irritants, and we become not a pearl but a person. We cultivate our hatreds, resentments, and revenge fantasies. We get hooked on potato chips, sales, saints, violence, soap operas, adrenalin, comic books, gold faucets, our appearance—hung up on some meat hook with our feet dangling above the ground, much of our freedom unavailable to us. We flail there, stubbornly unwilling or sadly unable to create the powerful manifesto for living that might begin to relieve a portion of our suffering. If you have read this far, isn't it time for you to create such a manifesto? Isn't it time to announce exactly how you intend to live, in pain perhaps but nonetheless proudly?

What might such a manifesto sound like? Here's one:

"My life is my project. Therefore I make certain efforts. I make these efforts according to my life purpose choices and in alignment with my values and principles. This is the high ideal I set for myself. As many times as I fall short of this ideal, that many times do I get back on my feet and return to my commitment. If I am plagued by thoughts that don't serve me, I work to get a grip on my mind. If I am plagued by behaviors that don't serve me, I work to extinguish them. If there is a deep sore spot in me, I work to heal it. If there is a wild, crazed place in me, I work to tame it.

"I know that I may have to change my circumstances, upgrade my personality, revise my worldview, seize new meaning opportunities, create new links in my causal chain, reach out for warmth and support, and much more. I will work to do all this. Unless there is some biological proof to the contrary—and I want to not only see that proof but also to be convinced by it—I do not accept that I have any sort of 'mental disorder or disease.' I may have anguish, terrors, rages, and more—but all of that is different from mental disease. I may even fall into some horrible holes out of which I can barely climb, but even then—even then—my life is my project. My pain is real, but so is my job of being human."

However you define your afflictions—as ADHD, PTSD, or OCD, as God's curse or the universe's indifference, as a bad draw or a failed effort—there is nothing except resistance that prevents you from creating your manifesto for living, living it, and seeing if some portion of your suffering vanishes as a result. To repeat, the mental health establishment has chemicals with effects to offer you, and you may want those effects. If a chemical "stabilizes your mood," "quells your anxiety," or "silences your voices," you may want those effects. But do not suppose for a minute that your job is done. You still have your manifesto to create and the project of your life to oversee.

However your society conceptualizes mental health and whatever it offers or refuses to offer by way of mental health services, you are obliged to separate yourself from its version and its vision. Can you do that? Can you dispute the contention of your tribal shaman that you are plagued by evil spirits if that is the village in which you grew up? Can you dispute the contention of your church elders that you are possessed by demons if that is the church in which you grew up? Can you dispute the contention of your psychiatrist that you have "clinical depression" if you grew up in a world revering doctors and medicine? The stakes are very high for you. If you can't, you may find yourself relying only on potions, exorcisms, or chemicals and not on yourself.

Because you are embedded in society, the future of your mental health is partly a function of how your society conceptualizes and deals with "mental health issues." If you would like to exert influence there and point your society in the direction you would like it to go, then that sort of activism and advocacy might well become one of your life purposes and meaning opportunities. I hope you see the matter exactly that way: I hope that you see the value in participating in the future of the mental health of our species. Your activism and advocacy are needed.

At the same time, you must look in the mirror. What do you want? Do you actually want to reduce your distress if that means that you must make changes? Do you want to stand up and make yourself proud by your efforts? I hope so. Then you are setting yourself real work. You will have to roll up your sleeves. Here comes a stale complaint that you have complained about a million times before. It needs banishing. Here comes anxiety rising up from some very deep place. It needs quelling. Here comes a spider's web of clever thoughts leading to apathy. It needs dismissing. Here comes a horrible memory. How will you survive it? Here comes a torrent of sadness. What will you do? These are your tasks. This is living.

Maybe you are one of the lucky ones who is not suffering that much, who has made peace with the indifference of the universe, who has found some work to love and some people to love, who finds life more fascinating than dreadful, who has a roof over your head and some treats in the cupboard and who can regularly laugh. Good for you! But I fear that I have some difficult news for you, too: please help others. Especially help the children. Our conception of the relationship between parent and child has changed over the millennia. If we have happily and luckily moved from a vision of children as chattel and farmhands, we have nevertheless slid into an odd new place of viewing them as proto-patients whose every behavior is a possible symptom of some mental disorder. If you are feeling pretty good, put your foot down for the children.

If you aren't feeling pretty good, there is no short answer as to what you might try, since the problem is life. It would be ridiculous to reduce the answers you need to items on a tip sheet. On the other hand, tips—like the tactics at the disposal of a human experience specialist—are not to be scorned completely. Here are a dozen that I think are worth your attention.

Twelve "mental health" tips:

1. Accept being human
    Human beings experience emotional distress in all sorts of ways: sadness, anxiety, addictions, unproductive obsessions, unwanted compulsions, repetitive self-sabotaging behaviors, physical ailments, conflicts of conscience, despair, boredom, and as all sorts of angry, bleak, and agitated moods. Can you accept this? Can you accept being human? When distress returns, can you stand unsurprised and, instead of blaming the universe, shrinking from the moment, or throwing up your hands, say, "I am a human being. I am nothing but human. Now, let me do what I can to gather myself and make myself proud!"
2. Acknowledge the straightjacket of personality
    Our personality is at once a pressure cooker and a windowless room. It sends our mind racing, it builds up grievances, it chooses sides, it frightens itself, it experiences disappointment and loss, it

maintains dark secrets, it gets violently aggrieved, it wants what it wants, and it knows how to hate at least as well as it knows how to love. Yet what it does and how it operates seem not to interest its owner. It is as if we are born with one genetic instruction before all others: "Never look in the mirror!" Your personality is your responsibility; your personality is your destiny. It may prove a terribly tight fit; only you can improve it.

3.   Be yourself

You must improve yourself—but you must also be yourself. This means asking for what you want, setting boundaries, having your own beliefs and opinions, standing up for your values, wearing the clothes you want to wear, eating the food you want to eat, saying the things you want to say, and in countless other ways being you and not somebody small or false. This doesn't mean denying the importance of others—of individuals, communities, civil society, and so on. Rather, it means that if you are gay, you are gay; if you are smart, you are smart; if you demand freedom, you demand freedom. Make use of your available personality to untwist the straps of your formed personality and be the person you intend to be.

4.   Invent yourself

You come with attributes, capacities, and proclivities, and you are molded in a certain environment. Your personality forms, and you become repetitive to a fault. But at some point you must say, "Okay, whatever is original to me—whether it's an extra dose of sadness, a bit too much sensitivity, whatever—and however I've been formed—to shrink, to fantasize, whatever—now *who do I want to be?*" You reduce your emotional distress by deciding to become a person who will experience less emotional distress: a calmer person, a less critical person, a less egoistic person, a more productive person, a less self-abusive person, and so on. You make the clear, conscious decision that, even as tightly wound as you find yourself, you will make use of your available personality and your remaining freedom to create yourself in your own best image.

5.   Love and be loved

Part of our nature requires solitude, alone time, and a substantial rugged individualism. But this isn't the whole story of our nature. We feel happier, warmer, and just much better, we live longer, and we experience life as more meaningful if we love and let ourselves be loved. We must be individuals, but we must also relate. To do both, to be ourselves and to relate, requires that we acknowledge the reality of others, that we not only speak but also listen, and that we make ourselves fit for relationships by eliminating our worst faults and growing up. If you have trouble loving, if you withhold, if you give yourself away, if you lead with criticism, if you can't get over yourself—whatever you do that harms your chances at love, remedying that ought to become one of your life purposes.

6. Get a grip on your mind

Nothing causes more emotional distress than the thoughts we think. We must do a better job than we usually do of identifying the thoughts that don't serve us, disputing them, demanding that they go away, and then substituting more useful thoughts. Thinking thoughts that do not serve you is the equivalent of serving yourself up emotional distress. Only you can get a grip on your own mind; if you won't do that work, you will live in distress. Think you are ruined? That thought will ruin you. Think you are unworthy? That thought will diminish you. Think the world is a cheat? That thought will disempower you. Your distress is not only held in firm place by the thoughts that you think, but it also *is* those thoughts. Imagine a day without inner commentary about everything that is hard, everything that is scary, and everything that is wrong. Wouldn't that be a better day?

7. Heal the past

We are not so completely in control of our mind, our emotions, or our being that we can prevent past sore points and the residue of trauma from returning with a vengeance. They have a way of pestering us as anxious sweats, as nightmares, as sudden sadness, and as waves of anger or defeat. They remain not only as memory, but as personality as well, woven into our fabric. But we can nevertheless try to heal the past by thinking through how we want to relate to the deep memories that are now woven into our fiber. What will you do when you are struck by a flashback? What tactics will you employ when you well up with rage or regret? From what reserve will you call up the energy to move through the pain? If healing is necessary then you must have tactics for healing, just as we need tactics to deal with epidemics. Healing is not a metaphor, it is a call to action.

8. Flip the anxiety switch off

Anxiety can ruin our equilibrium, darken our mood, and make all the already hard tasks of living that much harder. There are many anxiety management strategies you might want to try—breathing techniques, cognitive techniques, relaxation techniques, and so on— but what will make all the difference is if you can locate that inner switch that controls your anxious nature, flip it, and with that gesture flip on more calmness. With that one gesture you announce that you will no longer overdramatize, that you will no longer catastrophize, that you will no longer live a fearful life or create unnecessary anxiety for yourself. Anxiety is part of our warning system against danger, and by locating that switch inside of yourself and flipping it, you declare that you have decided not to live under siege and under threat. Threats remain, but flinging the chemicals of anxiety throughout your system is not really a helpful way to meet those threats. Being calm is better.

9. Make meaning

Our hardest lessons have to do with meaning. We do not understand that meaning is a "mere" psychological experience; we do not realize that adopting strong life purposes helps put meaning in its place; we have probably never thought through what are our exact personal requirements with respect to meaning. We can have much more meaning in our life if we stop looking for it, as if it were lost or as if someone else knew more about it than we did, and realize that it is in our power to influence meaning and even make it. By making daily meaning investments and by seizing daily meaning opportunities, we hold meaning crises at bay and experience life as meaningful. Meaning problems produce severe emotional distress, and learning the art of value-based meaning making dramatically reduces that distress. Learning this requires self-education, since nothing about meaning is taught in schools or by parents.

10. Let meaning trump mood

You can decide that the meaning you hope to make and the life purposes you intend to manifest are more important to you than the mood you find yourself in. Rather than saying, "I'm blue today," you say, "I have my business to build," or "I have my novel to write," or "I have my personality to upgrade." You start each day by announcing to yourself exactly how you intend to make meaning on that day, how you intend to deal with routine chores and tasks, how you intend to relax—how, in short, you mean to spend your day—and you consider all of that, the rich and the mundane alike, as the project of your life, one in which you are living with grace and in good spirits. You reduce your emotional distress by checking in more on your intentions and less on your mood.

11. Upgrade your personality

You may not yet be the person you would like to be or the person you need to be in order to reduce your emotional distress. You may be angrier than you would like to be, more impulsive, more scattered, more self-sabotaging, more undisciplined, more frightened. If so, you require a personality upgrade, which of course only you can supply. You embark on this upgrade by choosing a feature of your personality that you would like to upgrade and then asking yourself what sorts of thoughts align with this "upgrade" intention and what sorts of actions align with this "upgrade" intention. Then you think the appropriate thoughts and take the necessary action. In this way you become the person you would like to be, someone actually capable of reducing emotional distress.

12. Deal with your circumstances

Would you experience more distress relaxing at the beach or enduring a long jail sentence? Would you experience more distress if you hated going to work or loved going to work? Our circumstances matter to us. Our economic circumstances matter, our relationships matter, our work conditions matter, our health matters, whether our nation is at peace or is occupied by invaders matters. Many circumstances are completely out of our control, and many are within our control. We can change jobs or careers, we can divorce, we can reduce our calorie intake, we can stand up or keep quiet, we can do what we can do to improve our circumstances. As a result of these improvements, we will likely feel emotionally better. Reducing your emotional distress requires that you take real action in the real world.

These tips are of a self-help sort. The recent paradigm of self-help is completely available to anyone who would like to reduce his or her emotional distress. You can understand yourself, form intentions and carry them out, learn from experience, and grow and heal. Naturally, none of this is true if you are unwilling to do the work required. But if you are, you have an excellent chance of reducing your emotional distress and experiencing genuine emotional health.

Emotional health and pain-free living are not the same things. You can be as emotionally healthy as a person can be and still reel from the pain of losing a loved one, from seeing through the meaningfulness of your occupation, or from finding your intimate relationship falling apart. You can be as emotionally healthy as a person can be and still have real troubles every single day accepting your mortality, dealing with your lack of income, or tolerating your chronic pain. We must not judge emotional health by the amount of a pain a person experiences. A moral, mental, and emotional giant may be plagued by sadness; his opposite may be giddy with the pleasure of killing off the competition or acquiring some fine cigars.

What is emotional health, then, if it isn't the absence of pain? It is a kind of vibrant wisdom, a dynamic executive awareness coupled with a powerful resistance to humbug with a bit of philosophical wryness thrown in, a vibrant wisdom where you acknowledge your human nature and the facts of existence, see your life as your loving and deserving project, and live according to your life purposes and as a value-based meaning-maker. You are completely in the fray and just enough above it to see what the fray is all about. Does pain still arrive? Of course it does. You haven't learned how to walk on water—what you have learned is how to walk on fire.

I have been trying to make two points. First, there is a mental health establishment that is not doing a wonderful job of helping people in distress. The current establishment is dominated by a way of thinking that has fooled people into believing in the existence of "mental disorders and mental diseases treatable by psychiatric medication," when in fact the picture is completely different. I have tried to paint my own picture of what better mental health practices might look like. I have described a new helper, the human experience specialist, and outlined a repudiation of the pseudo-medical model of mental health services (with "chemicals with effects" still made available). I have proposed more and better thinking about huge questions concerning cause and effect in human affairs and the need for more and better institutions and communities of care. A paradigm shift really is needed—unless we are prepared to accept the inevitable outcome that soon virtually all children will receive one mental disorder diagnosis or another and will find themselves on powerful chemicals designed to suppress or relieve the symptoms of living.

Second, there is the challenging job that you have of maintaining your own emotional wellbeing and mental health. You will not get through life without emotional distress—a lot of it may be coming. That distress is already woven into you because of the way that personality operates like a straightjacket. That distress plays itself out in human ways like despair, hopelessness, and meaninglessness. It plays itself out through anxieties, addictions, manias, pestering obsessions, critical outbursts, and self-soothing indulgences. This landscape may demoralize you, but it had better not surprise you. Nothing prepared you for it—not your parents, not your schools, not your churches, not your leaders—and so you are obliged to understand your situation using your own wits and your own awareness. That is your starting point—then the work of personal mental health begins.

Suggested Reading

Barber, Charles. *Comfortably Numb: How Psychiatry is Medicating a Nation.*

Bass, Alison. *Side Effects: A Prosecutor, a Whistleblower, and a Bestselling Antidepressant on Trial.*

Basset, Thurstine and Theo Stickley. *Voices of Experience: Narratives of Mental Health Survivors.*

Bentall, Richard. *Madness Explained: Psychosis and Human Nature.*

Bentall, Richard. *Doctoring the Mind: Why Psychiatric Treatments Fail.*

Boyle, Mary. *Schizophrenia: A Scientific Delusion?*

Breggin, Peter. *Medication Madness: The Role of Psychiatric Drugs in Cases of Violence, Suicide, and Crime.*

Breggin, Peter. *Toxic Psychiatry: Why Therapy, Empathy and Love Must Replace the Drugs, Electroshock, and Biochemical Theories of the "New Psychiatry."*

Caplan, Paula. *Bias in Psychiatric Diagnosis.*

Caplan, Paula. *They Say You're Crazy: How the World's Most Powerful Psychiatrists Decide Who's Normal.*

Carlat, Daniel. *Unhinged: The Trouble with Psychiatry.*

Coles, Steven, Sarah Keenan, and Bob Diamond. *Madness Contested. Power and Practice.*

Conrad, Peter. *The Medicalization of Society: On the Transformation of Human Conditions into Treatable Disorders.*

Cordle, Hannah, Jerome Carson, and Paul Richards. *Psychosis: Stories of Recovery and Hope.*

Cromby, John, David Harper, and Paula Reavey. *Psychology, Mental Health and Distress.*

Fadden, Grainne, Carolyn James, and Vanessa Pinfold. *Caring for Yourself: Self Help for Families and Friends Supporting People with Mental Health Problems.*

Fancher, Robert. *Cultures of Healing: Correcting the Image of American Mental Health Care.*

Fisher, Seymour and Roger Greenberg. *From Placebo to Panacea: Putting Psychiatric Drugs to the Test.*

Geekie, Jim. *Making Sense of Madness: Contesting the Meaning of Schizophrenia.*

Greenberg, Gary. *The Book of Woe: The DSM and the Unmaking of Psychiatry.*

Healy, David. *Let Them Eat Prozac: The Unhealthy Relationship between the Pharmaceutical Industry and Depression.*

Healy, David. *Pharmageddon.*

Hornstein, Gail. *Agnes' Jacket: A Psychologist's Search for the Meanings of Madness.*

Horwitz, Allan and Jerome Wakefield. *The Loss of Sadness: How Psychiatry Transformed Normal Sorrow into Depressive Disorder.*

Johnstone, Lucy. *A Straight Talking Introduction to Psychiatric Diagnosis.*

Johnstone, Lucy: *Formulation in Psychology and Psychotherapy: Making Sense of People's Problems.*

Johnstone, Lucy. *Users and Abusers of Psychiatry: A Critical Look at Psychiatric Practice.*

Jones, Steven, Fiona Lobban, and Anne Cooke. *Understanding Bipolar Disorder: why people experience extreme mood states and what can help.*

Joseph, Jay. *The Missing Gene: Psychiatry, Heredity, and the Fruitless Search for Genes.*

Kinderman, Peter. *A Prescription for Psychiatry: Why We Need a Whole New Approach to Mental Health and Wellbeing.*

Kirk, Stuart, Tomi Gomory and David Cohen. *Mad Science: Psychiatric Coercion, Diagnosis, and Drugs.*

Kirk, Stuart. *Mental Disorders in the Social Environment.*

Kirk, Stuart and Herb Kutchins. *The Selling of DSM: The Rhetoric of Science in Psychiatry.*

Kirsch, Irving. *The Emperor's New Drugs: Exploding the Antidepressant Myth.*

Kutchins, Herb and Stuart Kirk. *Making Us Crazy: DSM: The Psychiatric Bible and the Creation of Mental Disorders.*

Laurance, Jeremy. *Pure Madness: How Fear Drives the Mental Health System.*

Levine, Bruce. *Surviving America's Depression Epidemic: How to Find Morale, Energy and Community in a World Gone Crazy.*

Maisel, Eric. *Life Purpose Boot Camp.*

Maisel, Eric. *Mastering Creative Anxiety.*

Maisel, Eric. *Rethinking Depression: How to Shed Mental Health Labels and Create Personal Meaning.*

Maisel, Eric. *Why Smart People Hurt.*

Moncrieff, Joanna. *A Straight Talking Guide to Psychiatric Drugs.*

Moncrieff, Joanna. *The Bitterest Pills: The Troubling Story of Antipsychotic Drugs.*

Moncrieff, Joanna. *The Myth of the Chemical Cure: A Critique of Psychiatric Drug Treatment.*

Rapley, Mark, Joanna Moncrieff, and Jacqui Dillon. *De-Medicalizing Misery: Psychiatry, Psychology and the Human Condition.*

Read, John and Pete Sanders. *A Straight Talking Guide to the Causes of Mental Health Problems.*

Rosemond, John and Bose Ravenel. *The Diseasing of America's Children: Exposing the ADHD Fiasco and Empowering Parents to Take Back Control.*

Ross, Colin and Alvin Pam. *Pseudoscience in Biological Psychiatry: Blaming the Body.*

Shannon, Scott. *Mental Health for the Whole Child.*

Shannon, Scott. *Parenting for the Whole Child.*

Shannon, Scott. *Please Don't Label My Child.*
Sinaikin, Phillip. *Psychiatryland: How to Protect Yourself from Pill-Pushing Psychiatrists and Develop a Personal Plan for Optimal Mental Health.*
Szasz, Thomas: *The Manufacture of Madness.*
Szasz, Thomas. *The Myth of Mental Illness.*
Tew, Jerry. *Social Approaches to Mental Distress.*
Timimi, Sami. *A Straight Talking Guide to Children's Mental Health Problems.*
Valenstein, Elliot. *Blaming the Brain: The Truth about Drugs and Mental Health.*
Watters, Ethan. *Crazy like Us: The Globalization of the American Psyche.*
Whitaker, Robert. *Anatomy of an Epidemic: Magic Bullets, Psychiatric Drugs, and the Astonishing Rise of Mental Illness in America.*
Whitaker, Robert. *Mad in America: Bad Science, Bad Medicine, and the Enduring Mistreatment of the Mentally Ill.*
Williams, Paris. *Rethinking Psychosis: Towards a Paradigm Shift in our Understanding of Psychosis.*

Index

Compeer, Inc., 146–47
connectedness, hope, identity, meaning, and empowerment (CHIME), 194

D

delusional mania, 161
depression
    antidepressant, 70, 72
    Barbara, 80
    biological cause lacking, 93–94
    childhood, 28, 90, 166
    clinical, 5, 43, 47, 71, 79, 127, 133, 159, 161, 176–77, 179, 201
    despair, ordinary, 199
    DSM and symptom pictures, 55
    Gould Farm therapeutic community, 146–47
    Jane, 176–77
    Jeanette, 83
    Jennifer, 87–88
    Jules, 82
    label, 93, 127, 159, 176–77
    "label" falsely implies that we know what is going on when we don't, 136
    life causes distress which causes "symptoms," 19
    life creates sadness and despair, 161
    life purpose and meaning, 74
    meaning crisis, 107
    mental disorder of, 22, 70, 72, 187, 199
    mental disorder *vs.* despair, 199
    mental health condition, 145–46
    Michael, 101–3
    mood-altering substance, 71
    "naming" alternatives, 126
    no biological cause, 93–94
    no reality to the term, 54–55, 192
    no such "disease" as, 192
    "normal" *vs.* "abnormal," 21
    psychiatric meds, 79
    psychological pain, 11
    Rachel, 85–86
    Sharon, 86
    "symptom" of, 133
    tag system, 177
    Tina, 84
diagnosis
    "anxiety disorder" diagnosis, 34
    of children, 43
    desire for relief without making changes, 38
    diagnose causes not the symptoms, 33

"diagnosing symptoms," stop, 42–43
"don't sweat the small stuff" training, 40
formulation of problem by the person, 39
human affairs, cause and effect in, 42–43
human experience, chemicals alter, 40
Jim, 34–39
Psychology Today article, 41
societal game of "diagnosing and treating mental disorders," 135
symptoms are not the diagnosis, 34
symptoms treated with time-tested tactics, 41
Diagnostic and Statistical Manual of Mental Disorders, Fifth Edition (DSM-5). *See also* Insel, Thomas; Szasz, Thomas
    catalogue for mental health professionals looking to make a profit, 54, 63
    catalogue of mental health labeling, xi, 56, 62–65
    causes of disorders, DSM is silent on, 56, 61
    "diagnose and treat mental disorders based on symptom pictures," 9, 54–56
    diagnostic manual that does not diagnose, 54
    fails to discuss causes, treatment, or prevention, 56, 63–65
    "manual lacks validity" (National Institute of Mental Health), 54–55
    medical-sounding justification for labeling people and for psychoactive chemicals, 55
    mental disorder definition, 58, 195
    mental disorders don't exist, 55
    psychiatric labels based on a symptom pictures, 61
    psychiatric/pseudo-medical approach, 192
    "statistical matter" lacking in manual, 60
    symptom is a medical condition *vs.* an indicator of a life situation, 63
    "symptom pictures" illegitimately become "mental disorders," 55, 60–62
    syndromes based on symptom pictures, 56
Diagnostic and Statistical Manual of Mental Disorders, Fourth Edition (DSM-4)
    mental disorder definition, 57–58, 195

uses heart, experiences, savvy, intuitions, and training, 123
uses tactics not taxonomies, 128
value, life purpose and meaning issues, 104–8
warmth and support, 148
"wise counsel" model, 186
human experiences. *See also* distress of life
about, 1–2, 8–9, 26, 39, 42–43, 56
Barbara, 79–81
calamity, 4
cause and effect, 89–98, 115, 134, 177, 182, 189–90, 207
chemicals with-powerful-effects, 76
DSM "symptom pictures" or "syndromes," 56
Jeanette, 83–84
Jennifer, 87–88
Jules, 81–83
motivation theories exclude, 1–2
Rachel, 85–86
sadness, 62
Sharon, 86–87
Tina, 84–85
human rights, 5, 13, 111, 137
humanistic theory of motivation, 3

I
incentive theory of motivation, 3
Insel, Thomas (National Institute of Mental Health), 54
insomnia
distress and, 91
epidemic, 5, 11
Jane, 172
job situation and, 91
Sally, 69–70
instinct theory of motivation, 3
institutional approaches, generally coercive, 192

J
Jane, 176–77
Jeanette, 83–84
Jeff (Philadelphia), 147
Jennifer, 87–88
Jewry, European, 2
Jim, 35–43, 50, 63–64, 70–71
John, 167–68
Johnny, 152–54

Journal of Consulting and Clinical Psychology, 46–47
Journal of Nervous and Mental Disease, 46, 167
Jules, 81–83
Jung, Carl, 8, 57, 63, 171, 174, 180, 195

K
Keropudas Hospital (Lapland, Finland), 140–41
Kirk, Stuart, 54–55

L
Laguna Honda Hospital (San Francisco), 142–44. *See also* Finnish Open Dialogue method
Laing, R. D., 8
Langer, Ellen (Harvard), 46–47
life coaching, 192
life formulation model
practitioner's relationship, 172–75
software program, 178–80
virtues of, 175–77
life purpose and meaning. *See also* distress of life; emotional distress; existential
about, 12, 74, 100–101, 106–8, 129, 132
human experience specialists, 106–7
life purpose boot camp classes, 107–8
meaning, creating, 108
mental health, future of, 105
mental health service provider, 100–101
Michael, 100–104
value-based meaning, 105
wellbeing, hedonic *vs.* eudaimonic, 105
Loyd (Anchorage, Alaska), 147

M
Mad in America, 137
Mad Science: Psychiatric Coercion, Diagnosis, and Drugs (Kirk, Gomery and Cohen), 54–55
manifesto for living, 201
Marcia, 179
marijuana, 68–69
marriage and family therapists, 186
meaninglessness, 5, 27, 167, 207
mental disease
biological bases of, 182, 192
distress of life *vs.*, 197
human distress, 197